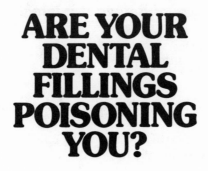

# ARE YOUR DENTAL FILLINGS POISONING YOU?

## Other Keats Books of Relevant Interest

THE ADDITIVES BOOK
by Beatrice Trum Hunter

BRAIN ALLERGIES
by William H. Philpott, M.D. and Dwight K. Kalita, Ph.D.

CANDIDA: A TWENTIETH CENTURY DISEASE
by Shirley S. Lorenzani, Ph.D.

DIET AND DISEASE
by E. Cheraskin, M.D.,D.M.D., W.M. Ringsdorf, D.M.D.
and J.W. Clark, D.D.S.

THE DO-IT-YOURSELF ALLERGY ANALYSIS HANDBOOK
by Kate Ludeman, Ph.D. and Louise Henderson

HOW TO SURVIVE MODERN TECHNOLOGY
by Charles T. McGee, M.D.

MENTAL AND ELEMENTAL NUTRIENTS
by Carl C. Pfeiffer, M.D., Ph.D.

THE NUTRITION DESK REFERENCE
by Robert Garrison, R.Ph. and Elizabeth Somer, M.A.

THE POISONS AROUND US
by Henry A. Schroeder, M.D.

TOXEMIA EXPLAINED
by J.W. Tilden, M.D.

YOUR BODY IS YOUR BEST DOCTOR
by Melvin Page, D.D.S.

# ARE YOUR DENTAL FILLINGS POISONING YOU?

## The Hazards of Mercury in Your Mouth– and What You Can Do About Them

Guy S. Fasciana, D.M.D.
with notes and a foreword by
Alfred V. Zamm, M.D., Lawrence M. Dickey, M.D.,
and William G. Crook, M.D.

Keats Publishing, Inc.  New Canaan, Connecticut

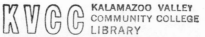

ARE YOUR DENTAL FILLINGS POISONING YOU?

Originally published by Health Challenge Press. Copyright © 1986 by Guy
S. Fasciana, D.M.D.

Keats Pivot Health Book edition published 1986. Reprinted by arrangement with the author.

ISBN: 0-87983-391-2
Library of Congress Catalog Card Number: 86-7348

Printed in the United States of America

Keats/Pivot Health Books are published by

Keats Publishing, Inc.
27 Pine Street (P.O. Box 876)
New Canaan, Connecticut 06840

## ACKNOWLEDGMENTS

A book is the mingling of a lifetime of ideas and experiences; not only of the author's, but those of the people who have touched his life.

I want to thank the physicians, patients and dentists who shared their thoughts and experiences with me in gathering the information in this book. Their contribution cannot be overstated.

Special thanks to Lawrence Dickey, M.D.; Kendall Gerdes, M.D.; George Kroker, M.D.; Donald Lombard, M.D.; Ann Nazzaro, Ph.D.; Victor Penzer, D.M.D., Dr.Med.; Theron Randolph, M.D.; and Alfred Zamm, M.D. for their suggestions and comments about the manuscript. I also want to thank Lester Hirsch, Ph.D., Western New England College, for his editorial help. Additional thanks to Harold R. Horn, D.D.S., author and Professor of Dental Materials Science, New York University, for his technical advice and expertise on dental materials.

Last and most important, I want to thank my wife, Terri, for her support and encouragement and for her help in writing and editing the manuscript, especially Appendix II.

Illustrations were done by Jill Atamian.

# TABLE OF CONTENTS

## CHAPTER ONE

**Human Physiology**

## CHAPTER TWO

**Toxicity**

# CHAPTER THREE

**The Immune System**

# CHAPTER FOUR

**Mercury**

# CHAPTER FIVE

**The Controversy Over Dental Mercury**

## CHAPTER SIX

### The Pro-Mercury Position

## CHAPTER SEVEN

### The Anti-Mercury Position

## CHAPTER EIGHT

### The Literature Review

## CHAPTER NINE

### Putting It Together

## CHAPTER TEN

**Surveys**

**CHAPTER ELEVEN**

**Amalgam Replacement: General Considerations**

**CHAPTER TWELVE**

**Amalgam Replacement: Special Considerations—
The Allergic and Environmentally Ill Patient**

## APPENDICES

# PERSPECTIVE

*By* ALFRED V. ZAMM, M.D.

Mercury toxicity: the problem was under our noses all along, and few people realized it! Of all the environments that have been examined ecologically, paradoxically it is the mouth that is the *last* to have been accorded the importance it deserves.

The relationship between preventable illness and the magnitude of the widespread endemic mercury toxicity from dental amalgam fillings has only recently become apparent. This recent observation resulted from a combination of the currently available better methods of measuring the presence of mercury together with the acute observations of practitioners.

In years to come, the controversy over mercury toxicity from dental amalgams and the numerous benefits that can be derived by its removal from the mouth will be compared to the controversy over the etiology of pueperal sepsis. Ignaz Semmelweis and Oliver Wendell Holmes fought so valiantly against stubborn opposition that denied the existence of germs as the etiology of pueperal sepsis. In retrospect, future generations will wonder why there was ever a controversy at all about removing a known toxin from the mouth, a toxin that never should have been put there in the first place.

Mercury toxicity is one of the major concerns of our time because mercury is a major toxin to which preventive medicine can be applied so successfully. This is one of the few situations in which a relatively easy application of preventive medicine can produce huge benefits.

This book is a wealth of valuable and difficult-to-amass information very useful to the dentist, the physician and the patient. It is a "how-to" book: how a dentist should practice, how a physician can make a diagnosis and how a patient can get well.

# FOREWORD

*By* LAWRENCE D. DICKEY, M.D.

Mercury toxicity or allergy from silver amalgam fillings should be suspected in those individuals who suffer from persistent ecologic illness and have not responded satisfactorily to dietary management and environmental control. A chronological dental history should be an integral part of the ecologically oriented medical history. Guy Fasciana, a dentist with knowledge and experience of ecologic illness, has written this book to help concerned patients evaluate their problems.

Dr. Fasciana first describes the physiology and immunology of how the human body responds to foreign excitants, whether toxic or allergic. Symptoms and injuries resulting from chronic mercury exposures are well defined.

Various diagnostic procedures and their shortcomings for evaluating the outgasing of mercury from amalgam fillings are discussed. In three chapters he proceeds to discuss the pros and cons of the mercury controversy emphasizing that there is no exact means of determining if mercury is a cause of the patient's problems.

The decision to remove and replace amalgam fillings is serious, expensive and controversial. The information in this book can help each individual make that decision. Once the decision is made, Dr. Fasciana describes the procedure to follow, which will minimize the exacerbation of symptoms during the replacement and the materials that should be used. Other substances used in dentistry such as nickel and acrylic have been reported to cause reactions in susceptible individuals.

Some dentists recommending replacement of amalgam fillings have extensive nutritional supplementation programs, which they prescribe before and after the procedure. This can and has resulted in unfortunate reactions. Dr. Fasciana agrees that nutritional supplementation should be under the direction of a clinical ecologist or physician who is aware of the patient's sensitivities.

Some enthusiasts would make it appear that controlling a mercury or *Candida* problem is the sole solution for the restoration of health. Both can be important factors in the management of ecologic illness, but are only part of the overall management and should be kept in proper perspective.

This book gives a well-balanced evaluation of the mercury problem which can be useful to the physician, dentist and patient in the management of ecologic illness.

## AN ADDITIONAL NOTE

*By* WILLIAM G. CROOK, M.D.

During the past two years two of my patients with yeast-connected illness, who had been improving on a comprehensive treatment program, experienced a sudden, major setback. In each patient a flareup in symptoms came after silver/mercury fillings were put in their teeth.

I've received similar reports from dozens of people who have written me. *So if I require fillings in my teeth, I'll ask my dentist to use something besides amalgam (silver).* Moreover, I now give my patients the same advice.

Recently I've been privileged to read the book *Are Your Dental Fillings Poisoning You?* by Guy S. Fasciana, D.M.D.. This carefully researched, easy-to-read book should interest you if you have silver/mercury fillings in your teeth.

You should read it if you're troubled by a chronic health disorder, including candidiasis . . . especially if you aren't improving on a comprehensive treatment program.

# INTRODUCTION

## A. HOW THIS BOOK CAME ABOUT

I remember a remark that a comedian made some years ago. He said: "If I knew that I would live this long, I would have taken better care of myself." At some point in our lives, we all decide to take better care of ourselves. I don't know if the reason for this interest is our desire for good health so that we can better enjoy life or if it is merely because we are afraid of getting sick. Whatever the reason, interest in our health is a positive influence on our wellbeing.

My "take-better-care-of-myself" time came when I got married. Both my wife and I were interested in cooking, gardening and health. Because of our interests and what we read about health foods, vitamins and healthful lifestyles, we made a commitment to eat properly, exercise and give ourselves the best chance to lead long, healthy lives.

In 1979, four months after moving my dental office into my house, I began to react to dust and pollen with the typical allergic symptoms such as nasal congestion, itching eyes and sneezing. These things never bothered me before; in fact, I never had any known allergies whatsoever. The "traditional" allergist that I went to at that time tested me for various molds and pollen and told me that, because I was allergic to dust, feathers and ragweed, I should avoid exposure to those substances.

During the next couple of years, I experienced an increase in my reactions to things in my environment. My symptoms expanded to include fatigue, food intolerance and weakness. I went to a specialist in internal medicine who couldn't find anything wrong. I later went to an endocrinologist (hormone specialist) at a well-known medical school who advised me that my symptoms were not allergy at all, but were due to low blood-sugar (hypoglycemia). He prescribed a five-hour glucose tolerance test. I was told that if the results of this test came back negative, he would want to do exploratory surgery, Needless to say, I was delighted to find that the test results were positive for hypoglycemia. The endocrinologist recommended a diet that consisted of six small meals a day. This new diet not only didn't solve my problems, but added to my food allergies.

In a short period of time, my symptoms expanded to include reactions to chemicals. Ultimately I became what is known as a "universal reactor." Universal reactors are people who have adverse reactions to most things in their environment. My adverse reactions included physical, neurological and psychological symptoms when I was exposed to chemicals and/or dental materials.

When I learned about my allergies to dental materials, I terminated my dental practice.

My attempt to avoid all the environmental substances which were producing these reactions was not entirely successful. There were still some things such as building materials (e.g., carpet, paint, particle board) that continued to provoke symptoms. I made a decision to purchase an "ecology trailer" which was built from stainless steel and porcelain and park it in the Pocono Mountains (Pa.). Living in the trailer enabled me to avoid the pollution of the city as well as other offending environmental substances.

During my stay in the trailer, my physician and I explored all known possibilities which could make me well again. Among these possibilities were avoidance of as many chemicals as possible (pollution, insecticides on food and chemicals), a special diet to minimize food allergies, medication for a Candida infection, immunotherapy for dust, mites, molds and pollen, supplementation for metabolic deficiencies and biofeedback. In addition to this treatment plan, my physician suggested that I look into the possibility that dental mercury could be contributing to my allergies.

Following his suggestion, I read several articles about dental mercury that had appeared in the *Journal of the American Dental Association* (JADA), but I remained unconvinced that mercury could be contributing to my allergic state.

The next year, I joined H.E.A.L. (Human Ecology Action League) and shortly thereafter, was asked to write an article about allergy to dental materials. I wrote four articles about dental materials. After the articles were published, I had quite a few readers write to me and ask about the mercury in dental amalgam fillings.

Knowing that there were some dentists who believed that the mercury in dental amalgam fillings could be harmful, I decided to investigate the validity of their opinions.

I knew that I could research the scientific literature and obtain testimony from physicians, patients and dentists in order to evaluate this question objectively. If it turned out that mercury was not a problem, that would be O.K.; if it turned out that mercury was a problem, then I would learn something that would help to improve my own health.

In the spring of 1985, I was almost finished researching the scientific literature on dental mercury when letters started to arrive from physicians and patients who had had their amalgam fillings replaced. Because of what I learned from the literature and what I was hearing from these physicians and patients, I decided that I would make arrangements to replace my own amalgam fillings.

The results of this decision have been very favorable. I have more stress tolerance, am able to space more time between meals, have more mental and physical energy and a more positive mental attitude. It may take some time to regain food tolerances since this is related to enzymes, the immune system and general health. Five months after having my amalgam fillings replaced, my elevated T-suppressor cells are now within the normal range.

The mercury picture is not entirely complete. I decided to publish my findings now because there are many physicians, dentists and patients who desperately need to know what information is available *now* in order to make their decision on replacing dental amalgams. The future will bring more definitive scientific research on the effects of dental mercury on the immune system as well as its effect on the human organism, more research on the biocompatibility of other dental materials, a bigger selection of replacement materials and some additional feedback from scientists, physicians, dentists and patients about the mercury problem. At that time there will be a new group of patients who will need new information to make their decisions.

This book is my effort to present the mercury dilemma as it exists today.

## B. PURPOSE

Where does mercury fit into the multitude of disease-causing substances? We know that man is able to adapt to most substances in his environment. There are times, however, when exposure to certain environmental substances leads to adverse (maladaptive) reactions. These reactions may be manifested through physical or psychological symptoms such as allergies, asthma, depression and fatigue. Some experts feel that maladaptive reactions might be the result of a body which is no longer able to cope with its environment. If this theory is correct, disease may be the result of a series of maladaptive responses. Therefore, it would make sense for us to minimize the unnecessary stresses that we place on ourselves in order to enjoy the benefits of health.

The dental office contains many materials such as denture acrylic, anesthetics and filling materials which are capable of causing adverse reactions. There are published case histories which have accused denture base materials (denture acrylic) of causing headache, rash, decreased grip strength, and increased pain in arthritic patients.[1] Of the dental materials which may cause adverse reactions, the safety of mercury (in amalgam fillings) is the subject of continuing controversy. This does not mean, however, that mercury is the *only* dental material of concern to the allergic (hypersensitive) patient or concerned dental consumer, but it is the material currently being implicated as the cause of various diseases.

This book focuses on mercury's role in disease: whether mercury plays no role in disease, whether mercury causes disease, or whether mercury acts in concert with other environmental factors to overload the body's biological systems and thereby cause disease. In order to assess the possible role that mercury plays in causing disease, we must understand how the body functions and how toxins can interfere with that function. This book incorporates current medical and dental knowledge about the effect that mercury may have on your body. It evaluates both the literature (scientific research) and clinical experiences of dentists, physicians and patients to enable you to have a more comprehensive understanding of the role that dental materials play in disease.

In attempting to meet the information needs of dentists, physicians and patients who will read this book, I found myself in a dilemma. How would I present enough technical information to satisfy the reader who has a background in the biological and chemical sciences and, at the same time, make the material understandable for the reader with no such background? The result is a technologically comprehensive discussion with in-text explanations where needed.

Don't be alarmed if Chapter Three, The Immune System, and Chapter Eight, The Literature Review, are difficult to read. This book is intended to be complete without your fully comprehending all the concepts presented in those two chapters. I have included a glossary of terms in Appendix I which lists the important terms discussed throughout the book.

Among the topics discussed in this book are:

1) The Physiology of Man
2) The Sources of Mercury Exposure
3) The Chemistry and Biochemistry of Mercury and Its Compounds
4) The Absorption of Mercury Compounds into the Body
5) The Chemical Changes Mercury Undergoes in Vivo (in the Body)
6) The Effects Mercury Compounds May Have on the Various Human Cell, Tissue and Organ Systems
7) The Mechanisms That the Body Uses to "Neutralize" the Effects of Toxins
8) The Controversy Concerning Mercury and Health
9) The Evaluation of Dental Mercury
   a) The Biological Effects of Mercury of Concern to the Patient
   b) Alternative Filling Materials
   c) The Methods for Amalgam (Silver Filling) Replacement

The purpose of this book is fourfold: to provide you with an understanding of human physiology, to evaluate the pro- and anti-mercury positions, to objectively present information contained in the scientific literature about dental mercury, to evaluate the alternative filling materials, and to provide you with feedback from patients, physicians and dentists about their experiences with dental amalgam replacement.

## C. THE CONTROVERSY OVER DENTAL MERCURY

Dentistry can truly be called an art. It involves both skill and creativity in the development of an aesthetic dental product. As with any art, the paths which lead to that finished product differ. Dentists have often disagreed about the best methods or materials to use for various dental procedures. Differing viewpoints have led to improvements in health care which have helped you and other patients. Most dentists are more than willing to share their "better way to do it" methods with both their colleagues and their patients. This informal learning process has allowed for improved dental treatment.

Dentistry is also a science because it develops principles based on a systematic collection of data through formulating, testing and drawing conclusions about dental health. Since most dental scientists are not practicing dentists, the scientific area has been more stable in its body of knowledge. Because of this stability, there has been broad agreement within the dental community about the scientific part of dentistry. The notable exception to this rule is the controversy concerning the safety of dental mercury. Since the introduction of amalgam to dentistry, its safety has had mixed reviews. This controversy continues today.

The issues raised by the pro-mercury and anti-mercury groups concerning the safety of dental mercury have resulted in confusion among health conscious consumers. Many patients are uncertain about their fillings and the materials used in them. They can no longer take their fillings for granted. In addition, our expanding knowledge and your concern over the safety of other dental filling materials will play a more prominent role in the future of dental treatment.

What I have done in this book is to provide you with the information you need to evaluate the safety of your fillings. Your first task will be to learn about human physiology; to understand how the "normal" human body should function. After this, you will be able to evaluate the conditions under which materials, such as mercury-containing alloys or plastics, can interfere with this normal human functioning. You will learn how the immune system protects the body from toxins and other foreign substances and evaluate the effects that mercury and other substances could have on this defense system. After you have learned about your body, you will be better able to evaluate what adverse effects fillings can have on your health.

Since there has been much controversy about the use of mercury in dentistry, this book will focus mostly on that subject. Other dental materials will be discussed later in the chapters on mercury-free filling materials.

If there was a definitive answer to the question about the safety of dental mercury, there would be no controversy. The difficulty in giving a definitive answer lies in the fact that there is no "normal" human being. Normal refers to a statistical average which does not describe you, the individual. What you must determine is "what is normal for you." In order to do this, you have to understand when your body is functioning normally and know what can interfere with that normal function. Basic to this discussion is the concept of health itself. You must decide, for yourself, when you feel unhealthy.

> Does healthy mean being free from a labeled disease such as hypertension?
>
> Must you have a diagnosed disease such as a diabetes to be unhealthy?
>
> Can disease include the beginning stages of a nutrient or enzyme deficiency; or, must there be signs and symptoms of a medically recognized disorder?
>
> At what point does health stop and disease begin?

After reading the material contained in this book, you will be able to apply *your* concept of health to each of the positions on mercury. You will be able to evaluate whether the mercury from your dental fillings can poison you and if you can be allergic to your dental fillings. At that point, you will be able to make a decision on what you want to do about your dental fillings.

## REFERENCES

1. Kroker, G., Marshall, R. and Randolph, T.: "Acrylic Denture Intolerance in Multiple Food and Chemical Sensitivity," *Clinical Ecology*, 1:48–52, (Spring) 1982.

# ARE YOUR DENTAL FILLINGS POISONING YOU?

# 1
# HUMAN PHYSIOLOGY

LOOKING AHEAD

1. BACKGROUND
   A. Your Body
   B. Vital Elements
   C. The Function of the Human Body
   D. The Essential Food Groups

2. THE NUTRIENT CYCLE
   A. Digestion
   B. Synthesis
   C. Excretion

3. WHAT CAN GO WRONG?

4. OVERVIEW OF PHYSIOLOGY

LOOKING BACK

# LOOKING AHEAD

The complex processes that occur within your body are mind boggling. Have you ever thought about what your body does with the food you eat? Your digestive system is like an assembly line; each part along the route has a distinct function in breaking down food and preparing it for absorption into your body. After each part does its thing, the goal of digestion is reached. What is this goal? The goal of digestion is to make the food you eat absorbable by breaking it down with enzymes into simple chemical compounds (amino acids, fatty acids and sugars). The body then uses these simple compounds, known as nutrients, for growth, repair, maintenance and protection.

Of course, a malfunction along the assembly line of digestion could cause an incomplete breakdown of food or decreased absorption of one or more of these important nutrients. A deficiency of any of these compounds would result in a breakdown of your biological systems which could make you more susceptible to illness. If your body is not efficient in using these vital nutrients, it will be more difficult for you to adapt to your environment—you will be "building-block" poor. Since nutrients are the building-blocks which your body uses to handle the stresses of daily living, a lack of building-blocks means that you are less adaptable. Although your body is versatile, there is a point beyond which adaptability is no longer possible; you must adapt or become a victim of your environment.

This chapter presents information on how your body gets nutrients from the food you eat, what your body does with those nutrients and what can interfere with your health.

# 1. BACKGROUND

## A. Your Body

Anatomically, man is divided into parts (organs), sub-parts (tissues) and sub-sub-parts (cells), each of which has a specific task to perform; all these parts together allow for the harmonious functioning of the human body. Cells form the structural basis of all plant and animal life. Each cell performs a very specific function. One such specific function is that of the red blood cell which carries oxygen from your lungs to all other cells throughout your body. Your tissues are comprised of groups of many similar cells; bone is a tissue. Tissues perform complex activities; the main functions of bone are to provide support and to maintain the proper concentration of minerals in your body. An organ is a group of highly specialized tissues. Your heart, for instance, is composed of specialized muscle tissues; its function is to rhythmically pump blood throughout your body.

To coordinate the activities of these various organs, your body has devised signaling systems. Distant cells, tissues and organs communicate with each other by sending chemical and electrical messages through your circulatory system and through your nervous system. By using electrical discharges, chemical transmitters and chemical reactions, your brain can reason, can recognize familiar faces, and can even tell your big toe what to do. When all your systems are performing in harmony, your body is said to be in balance and a state of health exists.

### B. Vital Elements

Essential to all life functions are air, water and food. The air we breathe contains oxygen which is necessary for respiration. The process of respiration involves supplying your body with oxygen necessary for metabolism and removing carbon dioxide, which is the waste-product of metabolism. This respiratory cycle is carried out not only in your lungs, but it is also an essential process in every cell, tissue and organ in your body.

Water is the medium which your body uses to carry out all life processes; it is also necessary for all internal activities. It enables nutrients to circulate and nourish all your cells; it provides for the excretion of waste-products and serves as the medium in which all chemical activity occurs.

Both pollution-free air and water, which are free of contaminants, are essential to carry out your necessary life processes without over-stressing your body. "Pure" food, i.e., food without added chemicals, pesticides, drugs or hormones, is also necessary for you to achieve and maintain optimum health. *It is obvious that the quality of your life is determined by the quality of the food you eat, the water you drink and the air you breathe.*

### C. The Function of the Human Body

The human body has three main functions: it builds new cells to replace those cells which have worn out; it repairs and maintains the working cells; and it protects the tissues and organs from injury and death. Some cells, such as red and white blood cells, can easily be replaced; certain tissues, like the skin, are also normally replaced or repaired without difficulty. On the other hand, there are cells so specialized that they can neither be repaired nor replaced. For example, your brain cells cannot be replaced if they die.

Protecting your cells and tissues is the responsibility of your immune system. This system recognizes foreign substances, such as bacteria and toxins, as being harmful to your body. It then mobilizes your white blood cells to attack, disable and digest these foreign substances. These white blood cells are our body's first line of defense. More complex defenses, such as antibodies, are used to protect our body once our white blood cells have begun the attack.

This process may sound simple, but it is so complex that we may never fully understand exactly how our bodies work. There are some things we do know. The experts have found that in order to carry out these vital functions, our bodies need certain nutrients contained in the air we breath, the water we drink and the foods we eat.

### D. The Essential Food Groups

Food contains three major nutrient groups: carbohydrates, fats and proteins. Carbohydrates are chemical compounds containing the elements carbon, oxygen and hydrogen. This is the general name given to all sugars and starches. Carbohydrates give your body a ready source of fuel for energy and supply some "essential" and "non-essential" nutrients. (Although we sometimes refer to nutrients as being essential and non-essential, *all* nutrients are necessary for life. If your body cannot manufacture a nutrient, physicians refer to that nutrient as essential. That is, your body has to be directly supplied with that nutrient either as a food or as a supplement. An example of an essential nutrient is vitamin C. Since your body cannot manufacture vitamin C, you must obtain it in the food you eat or through supplements. Non-essential nutrients are those nutrients which can be made from raw materials in your diet. An example of this is the conversion of carotene to vitamin A. Carotene is the substance found in yellow, orange or red fruits and vegetables such as carrots and apricots).

In addition to carbohydrates, fats provide a source of energy, as well as essential fatty acids which are used as parts of the membranes surrounding the cells (cell membranes). Fatty acids contain carbon, hydrogen and oxygen, but they differ from carbohydrates because of the arrangement (of the parts—atoms) of their molecules.

Finally, proteins provide the essential and non-essential amino acids that our bodies use to make antibodies, enzymes, hormones, and other proteins. Amino acids are compounds which contain carbon, oxygen, hydrogen and the $NH_2$ group.

Since there is no one food which contains all the essential nutrients, we should eat a variety of foods in order to get all the nutrients we need. A meal normally contains a combination of the three major food groups. For example, at breakfast you may eat eggs, toast, and fruit juice. Eggs provide you with protein and fats, and wheat provides mainly carbohydrates but also provides a small amount of protein and fat. Fruit juice contains carbohydrates which supply you with quick energy. These nutrient food groups provide you with the basic building-blocks in addition to vitamins and minerals your body uses for growth, maintenance, repair and protection.

## 2. THE NUTRIENT CYCLE

### A. *Digestion*

Digestion is the process by which our bodies break down the food we eat into amino acids, fatty acids and sugars. Digestion takes place in two ways: mechanical and chemical. The mechanical process begins with cutting your food into bite-size portions. Following this is chewing which breaks your food down into even smaller pieces. The purpose of chewing is to produce pieces of food small enough for your digestive aids (enzymes and hydrochloric acid) to divide them further. The chemical process includes digestive aids which break down foods into their simplest compounds. These digestive aids are produced in the mouth, stomach, pancreas, liver and the lining of the intestine (intestinal mucosa). Microorganisms found in the gastrointestinal (GI) tract also aid digestion.

During chewing, salivary glands, found in your mouth, produce enzymes which begin to digest carbohydrates. Your stomach secretes both enzymes and hydrochloric acid which help break down proteins and allow other enzymes to work. Your pancreas, liver and intestinal mucosa provide enzymes which continue the digestive process. Microorganisms produce acids and manufacture certain vitamins. This digestive process converts food into building-blocks of amino acids, fatty acids and sugars. These building-blocks are what your body needs for growth, repair, maintenance and defense. When you eat a variety of nutritious foods and your digestive system is working properly, you are able to get all the nutrients you need to be healthy. On the other hand, if you do not eat the proper foods or do not have the necessary enzymes, or your lifestyle and environment demand a greater amount of nutrients than you are providing for your body, illness is likely to follow.

The following chart summarizes the food groups and their respective components:

| Food Groups | Vital Nutrients Provided |
|---|---|
| Carbohydrate | Sugars |
| Fats | Fatty acids |
| Proteins | Amino acids |

## B. Synthesis

After foods are broken down into their simplest components, they are then absorbed into your body. Once these amino acids, fatty acids and sugars are absorbed into your body, your circulatory system distributes them to the areas where they are required for growth, repair, maintenance and protection. Some excess nutrients are stored in your liver and your bones until needed; others are excreted.

Synthesis is the combination of simple substances to form more complex compounds. Think of synthesis as putting together pieces of a puzzle to form a picture. You will assemble each of the individual parts (amino acids, fatty acids and sugars) to form a picture (proteins, fats and carbohydrates). Each picture has a role in either growth, repair, maintenance or protection. In the formation of the protein picture, amino acids are combined (synthesized) to form new proteins such as enzymes, hemoglobin and hormones. The new combination of these amino acids formed by your body is *your* protein; your "own brand." Your own brand of protein is different from the protein that was contained in the food you ate. For example, when you eat a chicken leg, you digest the chicken protein into its individual parts (amino acids) and then reassemble those parts into your own arrangement of amino acids to form your "own brand" of protein. It is important that you realize that your "own brand" of protein is different from the protein in the chicken that you ate. Your "own brand" of protein is also different from any other person's individual brand of protein, because your arrangement of amino acids differs from their arrangement of amino acids. Your body recognizes your "own brand" of protein as part of itself. I will refer to your proteins as "self" proteins, i.e., your "own brand" of protein. These "self" proteins are different from "non-self" proteins (foreign proteins) which are contained in the food you eat, such as beef, eggs and chicken. The proteins contained in foods are beneficial because the body can break them down into individual amino acids. However, foreign proteins in the form of bacteria and viruses are harmful because they pose a threat to your health.

Although we have been discussing protein synthesis, fatty acids follow a similar process. The new products which are synthesized from fatty acids are fats. Carbohydrates, after they are broken down into their component parts (sugars), are then either used for energy or are synthesized into larger carbohydrate units (glycogen) for storage.

| Food Group | End Product of Digestion | Product of Synthesis |
|---|---|---|
| Carbohydrate | Sugars | Glycogen (carbohydrate) |
| Fat | Fatty Acids | Fats |
| Protein | Amino Acids | Protein |

The process of digestion and synthesis is very complex and delicately balanced. If something goes wrong in this cycle, your entire system will suffer because you will be denied the essential nutrients necessary to complete your puzzle and remain healthy.

### C. Excretion

### 1) GENERAL EXCRETION[1]

Your cells produce waste products during biological activities. For example, carbon dioxide is produced from respiration, and uric acid and ammonia are produced from the breakdown of protein. You must efficiently dispose of these waste products. The process of getting rid of waste products is called excretion.

Excretion is accomplished through the lungs, the liver, the GI tract, the kidney and the skin. Ordinarily, your body can easily handle the removal of these products. In cases where the body cannot handle waste elimination (e.g., kidney disease, lung disease), those waste products accumulate in amounts that are toxic to you.

The initial step in getting rid of these waste products is their metabolism; that is, they are broken down to simple chemical compounds. Next, these simple chemical compounds are removed from your body through your lungs by breathing, through your liver which excretes them into the bile, through your GI tract in the feces, through your kidneys by urination and through your skin by perspiration.

A similar sequence occurs when your body eliminates toxins to which you are exposed. The toxins are metabolized either by enzymes in your blood plasma or by enzymes in your liver. White blood cells also help in this process. The chemical compounds are then excreted through your lungs, liver, GI tract, kidney and skin as were the waste products of metabolism.

Your lungs are a good example of this process. When you breathe, you inhale oxygen which is circulated by your blood to all parts of your body. In using oxygen, your body produces carbon dioxide as a waste product. Carbon dioxide is then transported to your lungs to be exhaled (excreted). Your lungs also excrete other gases produced by your body (e.g., ammonia) following the same process. As you will see later, mercury vapor may enter your body through breathing and much of it is excreted by your lungs.

2) THE ROLE OF THE LYMPHATIC SYSTEM

You are probably very familiar with your blood circulatory system, which consists of your heart and blood vessels (arteries, veins and capillaries), but you may not be as familiar with another circulatory system called the lymphatic circulatory system. The fluid (called lymph) in this system performs the function of removing waste materials given off by your cells and tissues. At strategic places along the lymph vessels are small "organs" called lymph nodes. These lymph nodes contain white blood cells (B-cells and T-cells) that respond to toxins and infectious agents. When your doctor tells you that you have "swollen glands," he is referring to swollen lymph nodes.

The process through which the cell's waste products are removed from the body include 1) cells and tissues give off waste products, 2) these waste products are dissolved in the lymph surrounding the cells and tissues, 3) the lymph circulates through the spaces surrounding the cells and tissues and enters the lymphatic vessels, 4) the lymph then flows through the lymph nodes where the T-cells and B-cells can respond to any toxins or infectious agents and 5) the lymph is then deposited into the general blood circulation to be transported to the liver and the kidneys for final disposal. (More about white blood cells in Chapter Three, The Immune System.)

## 3. WHAT CAN GO WRONG

The above examples were used as illustrations to explain complex processes which occur in your body. Each of the millions of reactions constantly taking place in your body needs specific raw materials. As we have discussed, some of these necessary raw materials are vitamins, minerals, amino acids and fatty acids. You need some additional compounds such as enzymes to help bring about the reactions.

Large or chronic interference can disable your system in any of the following ways:

1. MALABSORPTION—The malabsorption of nutrients can occur either through the improper breakdown of food because of a lack of digestive enzymes or faulty enzymes. Malabsorption can also be caused by diseases, such as inflammatory bowel disease, which can interfere with the absorption of nutrients. The net result of malabsorption is a deficiency of nutrients necessary to perform vital functions.

2. INCREASED DEMAND—Increased demand for specific nutrients may be caused by physical or psychological stresses. If a person is under physical stress caused by strenuous exercise or illness, certain nutrients will be in greater demand because the body will have to repair and maintain cells more quickly. Psychological stress also increases the demand for nutrients. For example, studies have shown that we need more vitamin C during times of stress. If there is an increased demand for nutrients and we want to remain healthy, we are faced with three choices: reduce the stress, increase the supply of nutrients or do both.

3. INEFFICIENCY—Your body is inefficient if it takes longer to complete or requires more energy to perform necessary functions. An example of this occurs when your body takes a long time to convert stored glycogen (carbohydrates) to simple sugars for energy. This delay in conversion may result in fatigue.

4. NUTRIENT LOSS—There are certain situations which promote the excretion of nutrients. Nutrient loss occurs when we excrete too much water. This can be seen with the use of water pills (diuretics) or in some diseases because minerals are excreted along with the water.

5. DRUGS AND CHEMICALS—Certain drugs and chemicals are capable of causing decreased absorption, increased demand or increased loss of nutrients, and would have a similar effect as outlined above.[2,3]

## 4. OVERVIEW OF PHYSIOLOGY

In order for your body to grow, repair, maintain and protect itself, you must supply it with and be able to use the essential nutrients found in air, water and food. Equally important is the efficient removal of waste products from your body. Your body takes food and breaks it down into its component parts (amino acids, fatty acids and carbohydrates). With these basic building blocks, as well as vitamins and minerals, your body then builds its own molecules (proteins, fats and carbohydrates). Some of these molecules are used immediately, while others are stored. Some of the carbohydrate is used directly for energy, and the excess is stored for later use. Some of the protein is used for growth and repair and some is used to manufacture enzymes that help chemical reactions occur. Protein may also make up hormones to help regulate your body or may form antibodies for protection, if needed.

A healthy body is an efficient body; it uses what it needs and stores the rest. As you have seen, there are many things which stress your system and may interfere with your health. The many steps that separate health from disease are difficult to identify. The body will go through many steps on its way from health to disease. If you pay attention to the signs and signals that your body gives you, you may become aware of this process. Listening to your body is an important part of staying healthy.

There is a wide range between the black and white areas of health and disease. In between these two areas is the gray zone of deficiency. This deficiency state gives rise to a variety of signs and symptoms. Health isn't an *all* or *none* phenomenon: today adequate nutrients; tomorrow disease. Generally, illness occurs slowly, and recovery seems to occur even more slowly.

The gray area between health and disease sparks debate among professionals and patients alike and seeks to answer questions such as:

1. Is a deficiency of nutrients resulting in the incomplete functioning of the human body, a disease state?

2. Must there be signs and symptoms of disease for there to be illness?

3. Can the gray areas between health and disease be measured? Can you ever know where you are positioned on the health/disease scale?

4. With what level of health are you satisfied?

You must develop a philosophy of health before you formulate a decision about your dental fillings. Your plan of action can then be based on your philosophy of health and on the information presented in this book. Your decision will depend on the state of health with which you are satisfied, what you are willing to do to achieve and maintain that state of health and your evaluation of the mercury controversy.

## LOOKING BACK

1. Your body is composed of cells, tissues and organs which communicate and cooperate to maintain balance within your body.
2. Your cells, tissues and organs require certain nutrients for proper functioning. These nutrients include amino acids, fatty acids and sugars as well as vitamins and minerals.
3. The essential nutrients needed by your body are contained in the food you eat, the water you drink and the air you breathe.
4. One of the major stresses on the body is easily overlooked; that is, the purity and quality of our nutrient sources: air, food and water.
5. Proper functioning of your body is necessary for the efficient use of nutrients. The efficient use of nutrients, in turn, provides for proper functioning.
6. Proper functioning requires the assimilation of food (digestion and synthesis), and the prompt excretion of waste products.
7. Since it is not always possible to measure body efficiency, it may be difficult to know where you are positioned between health and sickness.

### REFERENCES

1. Saifer, P. and Zellerbach, M.: *Detox*, Houghton Mifflin Co., Boston, pp. 23–30, 1984.
2. "Clinical Nutrition: Focus on the 80's," Department of Rehabilitation Medicine, New York University Medical Center, November 17, 1982.
3. Ganong, W.: *Review of Medical Physiology*, Lang Medical Publications, Los Altos, California, pp. 414–421, 1983.

# 2
# TOXICITY

LOOKING AHEAD

1. BACKGROUND

2. TOXICITY

    A. Mechanisms of Toxicity
    B. Effects of Toxicity
    C. Acute vs Chronic
    D. Mercury Poisoning
        1) Acute Mercury Poisoning
        2) Chronic Mercury Poisoning
    E. Overview of Toxicity
    F. Overview of Mercury Toxicity

LOOKING BACK

## LOOKING AHEAD

During the twentieth century, industry has moved from mechanical technology which focused on efficiency to chemical technology which focuses on convenience. This transition has led to development of pesticides and chemical fertilizers to increase crop production, and has led to the use of nuclear energy and insulation to make us energy independent. Although these developments have met society's short-term goals, they have also produced harmful by-products. We often read about toxic waste dumps, polluted ground water, and homes and offices which have become chemically contaminated. Each of the chemical by-products produced through these developments has adverse effects on our bodies; and because these products have an adverse effect, they are known as toxins.

However, toxins include more than just those chemicals used in industry and agriculture. You may wonder, what is a toxin? A toxin is any substance which has an adverse effect on a living system. Besides chemicals, some materials necessary for health can also be toxic. For example, an excess supply of vitamins can produce adverse reactions. Taking too much vitamin A can cause fatigue, hair loss, nausea, headache and vomiting; excess vitamin D may produce muscular weakness, nausea, vomiting and dizziness; an overdose of fat-soluble vitamin E can elevate blood pressure. Some vitamins have greater toxic potential than others depending on their solubility in body fat (among other things). Vitamin A, being fat soluble, is more likely to cause a toxic reaction than vitamin C, which is water soluble and rapidly excreted. These examples demonstrate that there is another factor to toxicity: the degree of exposure. Therefore, toxicity (adverse reaction) is related to the toxic substance and the dose (amount) needed to cause the adverse reaction. In general, the higher the dose of a particular toxin, the greater the potential for toxicity.

Many substances can be toxic to the human body; even necessary nutrients taken in excess can be toxic. Additionally, waste products produced by your cells add to your toxic burden if your body does not excrete them efficiently. Your body continually strives for a state of equilibrium. Balance is the bottom line.

This chapter discusses the concept of toxicity, the effects of toxicity on your body and the symptoms associated with mercury toxicity.

## 1. BACKGROUND

The concept of toxicity can be confusing. This confusion results from the fact that when two individuals are exposed to the same toxic substance one may get sick, while the other will not. Because a toxic substance can enter the body, circulate and be excreted does not necessarily mean that it will result in injury or toxic symptoms. In order to be toxic, a substance must adversely interfere with the way your body normally functions. An adverse effect can be so subtle that you are not even aware of it. This can be seen when a nutrient is tied up in the digestive tract by a substance which prevents it from being absorbed. For example, in the case of excessive tea consumption, the tannic acid contained in the tea ties up (binds) iron and interferes with its absorption.[1] However, tea is not considered toxic during ordinary consumption. This leads us to this question: Would tea be considered toxic if a person consumed a *normal* amount of tea but something in the person's environment was also binding to the iron in that person's intestines and the combination resulted in an iron deficiency? Or would tea merely be a contributory factor in toxicity?

On the other hand, a substance can increase the excretion of a nutrient. For example, drinking alcoholic beverages increases the urinary loss of zinc.[2] Another example is eating a food containing boric acid—found in some imported canned foods—which combines with and causes excessive urinary loss of riboflavin (a vitamin). Each of these examples can result in nutrient deficiency.[3] Excessive habits such as these can result in illness if continued over a long period of time. Toxicity as well as other medical matters, also has some gray areas, as we discussed in Chapter One, Human Physiology.

## 2. TOXICITY

### A. Mechanisms

You have seen that for a substance to be toxic it must produce an adverse effect on your body. To have an adverse effect, the substance must disrupt normal function. There are several ways that a substance can do this:[4]

1) ABSORPTION INTERFERENCE—Interference with absorption occurs in one of two ways: first, a substance can tie up (bind) vitamins, minerals, amino acids, fatty acids or simple carbohydrates. This binding can either decrease the amount of nutrient that is absorbed or can prevent its absorption completely depending on the concentration of the substance and how strong a hold it has on the nutrient. Second, a toxin can change the way your cell covering (cell membrane) allows substances to pass through. Scientists describe this change as an alteration in cell membrane permeability. There are four possible reactions to the change in cell membrane perme-

ability: 1) nutrients within the cell can be prematurely released, 2) waste products within the cell can be retained instead of excreted, 3) excess nutrients can flood the cell, and 4) the membrane can prevent nutrients from entering the cell. Each of these reactions disrupts normal functioning and is, therefore, toxic.

2) INTERFERENCE WITH RESPIRATION—A toxin can interfere with the process by which your body takes on oxygen and gives off carbon dioxide. As you breathe you inhale oxygen into your lungs; when you exhale you release carbon dioxide. In the lungs, oxygen attaches to hemoglobin, the substance which carries the oxygen and carbon dioxide. A toxin may interfere with this process by attaching to the hemoglobin and taking up the space where the oxygen or carbon dioxide would have been carried. If a substance interferes with this oxygen-carbon dioxide-hemoglobin interaction it is toxic because it disrupts the normal supply of oxygen to and the removal of carbon dioxide from the cells.

3) INTERFERENCE WITH ENZYMES AND COENZYMES—If a substance interferes with enzymes or coenzymes (a helper-enzyme) either by preventing them from forming or preventing them from functioning, it is considered toxic. For instance, coenzyme A is involved in converting sugar to energy. When a toxin interferes with this reaction the result is lower energy production. This lack of energy will affect your whole system by decreasing the efficiency of all cells and may result in fatigue, lack of concentration and the impairment of the growth, repair, maintenance and defense functions of your body.

4) ADVERSE EFFECTS ON THE IMMUNE SYSTEM—The immune system consists of cells, tissues and organs which defend the body against foreign substances. A toxin can interfere with your immune system by preventing your normal response to foreign materials. It can also mistakenly create a response to your own tissues. A toxic effect on the immune system is probably the most significant adverse reaction because the immune system is the key to adaptation. If a toxin prevents adaptation, then illness is inevitable.

### B. Effects of Toxicity

A toxin can produce both reversible and irreversible effects on your body. A reversible toxic effect means that the injury produced by the toxin can be repaired; an irreversible toxic effect means that the injury is permanent. The toxin's effect depends on its concentration, your cells' individual ability to regenerate and your susceptibility.

A toxin will cause more harm as its concentration is increased because, in higher doses, it injures more cells. In addition, the more complex the cell, the less able it is to regenerate. For example, injury to nerve cells is usually irreversible because these cells are highly specialized and cannot be replaced. Your skin, on the other hand, is less specialized and has the ability to be replaced. Therefore, a toxic effect involving your skin is considered less serious than a toxic effect on your nerve cells since your skin can regenerate and your nerve cells cannot.

As you saw in Chapter One, a toxin's effect varies with the individual. Some people are more efficient in counteracting (neutralizing) and eliminating toxic substances. Others have difficulty in neutralizing toxins. These people have more severe symptoms over a longer period of time. Toxic symptoms can occur anywhere in your body. They are not necessarily confined to the area (local type of reaction) where the toxin made contact with your body. An example of this systematic type of toxic reaction is a type of food poisoning known as botulism. Botulism occurs when meat, fruits or vegetables are not properly sterilized in canning. This results in an accumulation of toxins produced by certain bacteria. After eating the affected food, the person digests the foods and the toxins that were produced by the bacteria entering the circulatory system. These toxins act on the nervous system causing paralysis.

### C. Acute vs Chronic

There are two types of toxicity: acute and chronic. Acute toxicity occurs from a single large exposure to a toxin and results in easily identified signs and symptoms. Chronic toxicity occurs from exposure to small quantities of a toxic substance over a long period of time. This chronic exposure results in the accumulation of that toxin in your system. This *cumulative toxic effect* is most important because when a toxin accumulates in your cells, the toxic effects are prolonged. Chronic toxicity poses an added danger to your health. Because chronic toxicity is a gradual poisoning, you may never realize that you are being exposed to the toxin. Your symptoms may be so vague that you are not able to identify their cause. In reality, your body never has a chance to bounce back. This inability to recover further reduces your adaptability to other stresses in your environment and eventually results in disease.[5]

## D. Mercury Poisoning

### 1) ACUTE MERCURY POISONING

Although we have been using the word *toxin* to describe a substance which produces adverse effects on your body, we can also describe a toxin as a poison. Acute mercury toxicity is also described as acute mercury poisoning. Mercury can be found in three forms: elemental mercury, inorganic mercury and organic mercury. (The individual forms of mercury are discussed in Chapter Four.) Acute mercury poisoning can occur from any of these three forms of mercury.

First, poisoning can occur if an individual swallows inorganic salts of mercury such as mercuric chloride (calomel). Mercuric chloride is an ingredient of some skin creams. A symptom associated with swallowing mercuric chloride is an ashen-gray appearance of the lining of the mouth. This occurs because the protein in the lining of the mouth coagulates as protein does when you fry an egg. Additional symptoms are pain, vomiting, and diarrhea. Poisoning can also occur when mercury-containing skin cream is used.

The inhalation of mercury vapors can also cause poisoning. Mercury vapor is found in both mercury ore deposits and as a chemical agent in industry, chemistry laboratories and in the dental office. Inhaling the fumes of mercury results in an inflammation of the lungs, unconsciousness, elevation of temperature, cough, chest pain, dark coloring under the skin, diarrhea, vomiting, rapid breathing, decreased oxygen absorption by the lungs, breathlessness and bleeding.

Finally, mercury poisoning can result if organic mercury such as methyl mercury is swallowed. Methyl mercury is the form of mercury which has been found in some seafood. Methyl mercury is 100 to 1,000 times more toxic than any other form of mercury.

Symptoms from any type of acute mercury poisoning start within a few hours of swallowing or breathing the mercury. Oral symptoms include metallic taste, inflammation of the lining of the mouth, foul breath, sore gums, excessive saliva in the mouth and discoloration of the gums (gingival margin). Later symptoms in the mouth include local infection, loosening of teeth and irreversible damage to the jaw bone (necrosis of the alveolar process). Symptoms which affect the nervous system include unconsciousness, excitement, exaggerated reflexes, and involuntary trembling movements. When mercury reaches the intestines the result is an inflammation of the intestines (colitis). The kidneys react to acute mercury poisoning by increasing urination (diuresis) and preventing the reabsorption of nutrients.[6]

I have outlined the symptoms of acute mercury poisoning below. You should be aware that both mercury vapor and mercury salts cause the same symptoms. This is because mercury vapor is changed to mercury ions (mercuric ions) in the body and the body doesn't distinguish where the mercury ion came from.

*Outline of Acute Mercury Poisoning Symptoms*

*Oral Symptoms*
1. Lining of the mouth (mucous membranes) has ashen-gray appearance
2. Stomatitis—inflammation of the mucous membranes
3. Foul breath
4. Sore gums
5. Discoloration of the gums (gingival margin)
6. Metallic taste
7. Excessive salivation
8. Local infection—gingivitis (infection of the gums)
9. Loosening of teeth
10. Necrosis of the alveolar process—irreversible damage to the jaw bone

*General Physical Symptoms*
1. Oral pain
2. Vomiting
3. Diarrhea
4. Lethargy—deep and prolonged unconsciousness
5. Fever
6. Tachypnea—rapid breathing
7. Hemorrhage—bleeding

*Central Nervous System Symptoms*
1. Excitement
2. Hyperreflexis—exaggerated tendon reflex
3. Tremor—involuntary trembling movement

*Gastrointestinal Symptoms*
1. Colitis—inflammation of the colon (lower part of the GI tract)

*Renal Symptoms*
1. Diuresis—production of unusually large amounts of urine
2. Inhibited reabsorption of nutrients

*Symptoms That Indicate Inhalation of Mercury Vapor*
1. *Pneumonitis—inflammation of the lungs*
2. *Tachypnea—rapid breathing*
3. *Cough*
4. *Chest pain*
5. *Cyanosis—dark blue color of the skin due to the lack of sufficient oxygen in the blood*
6. *Atelectasis—failure of the lungs to absorb oxygen*
7. *Emphysema—breathlessness on exertion due to decreased oxygen absorption*
8. *Pneumothorax—presence of air in the chest cavity*

2) CHRONIC MERCURY POISONING

Chronic mercury poisoning occurs from the exposure to small amounts of mercury over a long period of time. It generally occurs as a result of prolonged exposure to any of the three forms of mercury. Neurological or psychiatric symptoms include depression, irritability, exaggerated response to stimuli, excessive shyness, insomnia, emotional instability, forgetfulness and confusion. Other neurological signs include spasms of the arms, legs or facial muscles (chorea), lack of muscle coordination, and mental retardation. Additional symptoms (vasomotor symptoms) found are excessive perspiration, uncontrollable blushing, and fine trembling of fingers, eyelids, lips, and tongue. Tremors may be minimal at rest and increase with stress. These symptoms are related to the concentration (dose) of toxin. At very low concentrations, symptoms are fewer and not as dramatic. As the concentration increases, the number and severity of symptoms increases.

As you have seen in acute mercury poisoning, both mercury vapor and mercury salts produce the same reaction. These exposures primarily affect the kidney. If the dose is high enough to cause toxicity, the symptoms which result are excess protein (proteinuria) but not excess amino acids in the urine, abnormally small amounts of protein in the blood (hypoproteinemia) and the accumulation of excessive amounts of watery fluid in the cells or tissues (edema). Other effects of chronic mercury toxicity include inflammation of the gums, inflammation of mucous membranes and excess saliva. Some non-specific symptoms include diminished appetite, weight loss, anemia and muscular weakness.

Chronic methyl mercury toxicity includes most of the same symptoms that are produced by mercury vapor and mercury salts. However, the kidney is usually not affected by methyl mercury. Pregnant women exposed to methyl mercury without having symptoms of toxicity have given birth to children who later developed cerebral palsy.[7]

Trakhtenberg[8] relates symptoms of chronic low-dose exposure to mercury (micromercurialism), first described by Stock,[9] as falling into three groups according to degree of intensity of the exposure:

> "First degree micromercurialism results in lowered working capacity, increased fatigue, light nervous excitability . . . in the second degree there is swelling of the nasal membranes, progressive weakening of memory, feelings of fear and loss of self-confidence, irritability, headaches. Simultaneously there may be catarrhal symptoms and upper respiratory discomfort, changes in the mucous membranes of the mouth, bleeding gums. Sometimes there are feelings of coronary insufficiency, shivering, quickening pulse, and a tendency towards diarrhea. The third degree micromercurialism is characterized by symptoms approaching those of regular mercurialism [acute mercury exposure], but to a lesser degree. The symptoms of this stage are: headaches, general weakness, sleeplessness, decline in intellectual capacity, depression. Among other signs are tears, diarrhea, frequent urination, a feeling of pressure in the cardiac region and shivering."

Below is an outline of the signs and symptoms of chronic mercury poisoning (micromercurialism).

### *Outline of Chronic Mercury Poisoning Symptoms*

Neurological or Psychiatric Symptoms
1. Depression
2. Irritability
3. Erthism—exaggerated response to stimuli
4. Excessive shyness
5. Insomnia
6. Emotional instability
7. Forgetfulness
8. Confusion
9. Chorea—irregular, spasmodic, involuntary movements of the limbs or facial muscles
10. Ataxia—uncoordinated muscular movements
11. Seizures—an attack. It may not be limited to convulsions.
12. Mental retardation

Vasomotor Symptoms
1. Excessive perspiration
2. Uncontrollable blushing
3. Fine trembling of the fingers, eyelids, lips and tongue

Oral Symptoms
1. Gingivitis—inflammation of the gums
2. Stomatitis—inflammation of the mucous membranes
3. Excessive salivation

Non-specific Symptoms
1. Pregnant women have given birth to children who developed cerebral palsy
2. Nephrotoxicity—toxicity of the kidney resulting in proteinuria (inorganic mercury exposure)
3. Anorexia—diminished appetite, aversion to food
4. Weight loss
5. Anemia—any condition in which the number of red blood cells, the amount of hemoglobin or volume of packed red blood cells is less than normal. Frequently manifested by pallor (lack of color) of the skin and mucous membranes, shortness of breath, palpitations of the heart, soft systolic murmurs and fatigue.
6. Muscle weakness

### E. Overview of Toxicity

As you have seen, any substance which adversely affects your body's functioning is considered toxic. The exposure can be acute or chronic; the effects can be subtle or dramatic; and the injury can be reversible or irreversible. An acute exposure is a single large toxic dose. Chronic toxicity results from exposure to small quantities of a toxin over a long period of time. Acute exposures usually produce dramatic effects because the toxin causes injury faster than the body can neutralize and excrete the toxin. On the other hand, repeated exposure to toxins (chronic exposure) produces symptoms which are more subtle because the body can more effectively dispose of the toxin but cannot completely eliminate it. The acute or chronic effects of the toxin can be either reversible or irreversible depending on the type of cell affected. Injury which cannot be repaired is irreversible, whereas injury which can be repaired is reversible. The more specialized the cell the more permanent the damage. If you are exposed to a high concentration of toxin, are not able to neutralize and excrete it, and the toxin interferes with cells which are specialized and cannot regenerate, the toxic effect will be dangerous and irreversible.

Some of the important ways that toxins can interfere with your normal functioning are through interference with absorption, interference with respiration, interference with enzymes or coenzymes and through adverse effects on the immune system.

### F. Overview of Mercury Toxicity

As with any toxin, toxicity to mercury can be acute or chronic. This will depend on the form of mercury, the concentration of mercury, the period of exposure, the number of different sources of exposure, the areas of the body affected and the individual's ability to neutralize and excrete the mercury to which he is exposed. Once it enters the body, mercury can combine with many compounds that are important to proper functioning. For example, mercury has a strong attraction for sulfur, nitrogen, oxygen and the halogens (chloride, bromide, and iodide). These elements are contained in compounds throughout your body. When mercury combines with one of these elements, it creates a powerful bond. It is because of this strong attraction and powerful bond that mercury is toxic. One of the most widespread elements in your body is sulfur. It is contained in compounds in virtually every cell and tissue in your body; it is part of certain amino acids, proteins, hormones, antibodies and enzymes. Let's look at an example. An enzyme is a helper molecule. By helper molecule, I mean that an enzyme causes a chemical reaction to occur without being used up in the process. Because it is not used up in the process, a small amount of enzyme can allow the same reaction to occur many times. If an enzyme involved in cell metabolism contains sulfur, and mercury binds with the sulfur, the result is that the mercury-sulfur combination prevents that enzyme from working. The mercury toxicity occurs because the enzyme is paralyzed by mercury.

The attraction that mercury has to these elements not only determines its toxicity but also forms the basis for treatment of mercury poisoning. It is because of this affinity for mercury that dimercaprol and penicillamine can be used to treat mercury poisoning. They will pull mercury out of the body by combining with it.[10]

Dental patients who are concerned that their amalgam fillings might be toxic should be concerned with *chronic toxicity* since their exposure to dental mercury is with a small quantity over a long period of time.

# LOOKING BACK

1. To be toxic, a substance must directly or indirectly interfere with one or more bodily functions. This interference can range from something basic like the interference with the absorption or excretion of a particular nutrient to the more complex disruption of an enzyme system.
2. There are several ways by which a toxic substance can disrupt normal functioning:
   A. Interference with absorption
   B. Interference with respiration
   C. Interference with enzymes and coenzymes
   D. Adverse effects on the immune system
3. There are two types of toxicity: acute and chronic. Acute toxicity results from a dose of toxin delivered as a single event; chronic toxicity results from a small quantity of toxin delivered over a long period of time.
4. Mercury poisoning can result from an acute or chronic exposure. Dental patients concerned with the adverse effects from the mercury in their amalgam fillings should be concerned with the chronic type of exposure to mercury.

## REFERENCES

1. "Clinical Nutrition: Focus on the 80's," Department of Rehabilitation Medicine, New York University Medical Center, p. 63, November 17, 1982.
2. *Ibid.*, p. 57.
3. *Ibid.*, pp. 17–21.
4. Gilman, A., Goodman, L. and Gilman, A.: *The Pharmacological Basis of Therapeutics*, Macmillan Pub. Co., pp. 1602–1628, New York, 1980.
5. *Ibid.*, pp. 1602–1603.
6. *Ibid.*, p. 1624.
7. *Ibid.*, p. 1625.
8. Trakhtenberg, I.: *Chronic Effects of Mercury on Organisms* (Translation by Fogarty International Center for Advanced Study in the Health Sciences), U.S. Dept of HEW Public Service, National Institute of Health, D HEW Pub (NIH) 74-473, 1974.
9. Stock, A., Z. *Angew. Chem.*, 39:461, 1926.
10. Gilman, A., Goodman, L. and Gilman, A.: *The Pharmacological Basis of Therapeutics*, Macmillan Pub. Co., p. 1623, New York, 1980.

# 3
# THE
# IMMUNE SYSTEM

LOOKING AHEAD

1. BACKGROUND

2. CELL FUNCTION

3. CELL FUNCTION SUMMARY

4. IMMUNE ENZYMES

5. IMMUNE PROTEIN FUNCTION

6. IMMUNE RESPONSES
   A. Humoral
   B. Cellular

7. WHAT CAN GO WRONG?

8. EXAMPLES OF IMMUNE MALFUNCTION

9. THE EXPANDED CONCEPT OF ALLERGY

LOOKING BACK

## LOOKING AHEAD

The main purpose of your immune system is defense. It defends you from invasion by foreign substances (toxins, bacteria, viruses). In order to protect you from these foreign substances, your immune system must first distinguish what substances are yours and what substances are not yours (foreign). In this respect, your immune system is like an "inspector general." The inspector checks out each item passing his way and puts that item into one of two groups: "self" or "non-self." The "self" group consists of your own cells, tissues and organs and their chemical compounds. The "non-self" (foreign) group consists of anything which the inspector does not recognize as a part of you ("self"). This system of recognition accomplishes two goals: it allows your body to protect itself from foreign substances and it realizes that your own body parts pose no threat to your safety. This monitoring device maintains the important balance necessary for you to stay healthy.

This chapter presents information about how your immune system works. I will discuss the parts of the immune system, how it distinguishes "self" from "nonself," the various immune responses and what can interfere with the immune system at work. The immune system is at the very heart of the mercury controversy because the anti-mercury group asserts that mercury in dental amalgam fillings causes diseases related to immune function. In deciding whether dental mercury is toxic to the body and, if toxic, whether this toxicity can interfere with the immune system, it is important to answer such questions as:

If mercury is toxic, can that toxicity impair the way your immune system recognizes your own cells or your own chemical compounds?

Can mercury toxicity alter the way your immune system reacts to substances which are foreign but not threatening (e.g., food)?

Can you be allergic to mercury?

If you can be allergic to mercury, can dental amalgam be a source of the mercury which is supporting your allergy?

## 1. BACKGROUND

The information about the immune system is complex and may be difficult to understand. I have tried to simplify the material as much as possible and at the same time provide you with an adequate background to be able to understand the effects of toxins on the immune system.

The immune system consists of cells, tissues and organs. The cells that make up the immune system are white blood cells which include B lymphocytes, T lymphocytes and macrophages. The tissues and organs which are part of the immune system are the thymus gland, lymph nodes, spleen and bone marrow. In addition to these cells, tissues and organs are specific plasma proteins (antibodies) and the plasma enzymes, complement. The purpose of the immune system is defense; that is to recognize foreign materials and render them harmless. It does this by recognizing harmful bacteria, viruses or toxins entering the body and rendering them harmless through a complex and delicately balanced series of interactions between white blood cells, plasma enzymes and specific plasma proteins.

## 2. CELL FUNCTION

Your blood contains three general types of cells: red blood cells, platelets, and white blood cells. Red blood cells transport oxygen from the lungs to all other tissues and transport carbon dioxide from those tissues back to the lungs. Platelets, very small disk-shaped cells, are involved in blood clotting. White blood cells are the defense center of your body.

There are three general categories of white blood cells: granulocytes, monocytes and lymphocytes. These cells provide your body with powerful defenses against tumors and infections. Granulocytes include neutrophils, eosinophils and basophils. The neutrophils seek out, digest and kill bacteria; they are your first line of defense against bacteria. Eosinophils attack some types of parasites and are involved in allergic reactions. Basophils participate in allergic reactions by releasing histamine. Histamine allows materials to pass in and out of your blood vessels more easily.

The monocytes also attack infections. They follow the neutrophils into the area of infection and are considered to be your second line of defense. Monocytes are converted into macrophages shortly after entering your circulatory system. These macrophages play a key role in your immune responses; they process antigen and "hand it" to the B-cells. Lymphocytes which include B lymphocytes (B-cells) and T lymphocytes (T-cells) are very important cells in your immune system, as we shall see shortly.

The white blood cells originate in your bone marrow. These white blood cells are formed from cells that have no specific identity (stem cells). Stem cells have the potential to become any of the different white blood cells depending on which type of white blood cells is needed. Let's take a closer look at the key players of the immune system: the B lymphocytes, T lymphocytes and macrophages.

B lymphocytes (B-cells) comprise 10 to 20 percent of your circulating blood lymphocytes. They produce specific proteins known as antibodies. Antibodies combine with only those substances that caused their formation. For example, a bacterium, which we will call bacterium "A," enters your body. Bacterium "A" contains specific proteins, called "A" antigens, which your immune system recognizes as foreign or "non-self." Your immune system then produces specific proteins called "A" antibodies. It sends these antibodies into the blood stream to find and attach to bacterium "A." The purpose of these antibodies is to combine with their antigens, to immobilize them, and to allow the other white blood cells to digest the antigen-antibody combination (antigen-antibody complex). Let's summarize what happens. "A" enters your body, your immune system recognizes it as foreign and produces "A" antibodies. "A" antibodies attach to the protein part of "A," immobilize it and allow other white blood cells to digest "A." The significant part of this story is that the antibodies produced by your immune system against bacterium "A" only work against bacterium "A." If, for instance, bacterium "B" should enter your body, new antibodies would have to be produced.

T lymphocytes (T-cells), mature in the thymus gland, and comprise 70 to 80 percent of the circulating blood lymphocytes. T-cells have many functions. Among the most important is to turn on and turn off B-cells. By turning B-cells on and off, T-cells regulate antibody production. There are four types of T-cells: helper T-cells (T4), suppressor T-cells (T8), activator T-cells and effector T-cells. The helper T-cells "help" B-cells. That is, they turn on B-cells to produce antibodies (when harmful bacteria enter the body). Suppressor T-cells turn off B-cells. That is, they curb the production of antibodies by the B-cells (as soon as a foreign substance has been rendered harmless). Activator T-cells "activate" other T-cells. They tell the helper T-cells and the suppressor T-cells when to work. Effector T-cells destroy foreign cells, such as bacteria, and are sometimes referred to as killer T-cells. You should be aware, that without T-cell control, B-cells cannot distinguish harmless substances (e.g., dust, pollen and foods) from harmful substances (e.g., toxins, bacteria and viruses). B-cells would react indiscriminately at an uncontrolled rate producing unlimited antibodies. This frenzied activity would result in a tremendous number of immune complexes (antigen-antibody combinations) which the body would have to process. It is the T-cells that keep these reactions in balance; and it is the balance (ratio) between the helper T-cells and the suppressor

T-cells that is crucial in keeping the immune system functioning properly. The T4/T8 ratio accepted as normal, ranges from 1.8/1 to 2/1.[1]

Macrophages, which mature in the tissues, have two responsibilities: they bring the foreign material (antigen) to the cells that are capable of producing antibodies and they digest (process) immune complexes. Immune complexes are combinations of antigens and antibodies. Macrophages digest the immune complexes into their component parts (proteins, carbohydrates and fats) and your body then excretes them (see Figure 1).

## 3. CELL FUNCTION: SUMMARY

| *Immune Cells* | *Function of Cells* |
|---|---|
| B-cells | Produce antibodies |
| T-cells | Regulate B-cells |
| Macrophages | Present antigen and process immune complexes |

## 4. IMMUNE ENZYMES

Beside the white blood cells, the immune system contains various enzymes which help the white blood cells to disable the antigen (foreign substance). These enzymes are collectively called "complement." Complement is the middleman which helps antigens (foreign substances) combine with circulating antibodies. This process results in breakage (lysis) of the foreign cells. Complement also aids in the attraction of white blood cells (leukocytes) to the antigen.

## 5. IMMUNE PROTEINS

Antibodies are special proteins (immunoglobulins) which circulate in the blood. As we discussed in Cell Function, above, these antibodies are produced by the B-cells. There are five general types of immunoglobulins: IgG, IgA, IgM, IgD and IgE. Each immunoglobulin consists of two chains of proteins; a long chain and a short chain. These two chains of proteins are joined by sulfur bridges (disulfide bridges).

To give you an example of how immunoglobulins work, I will discuss IgA. In the intestines, are microfold cells (M-cells) which take bacterial and viral antigens and pass them to special underlying tissue (lymphoid tissue). The antigen stimulates cells (lymphoblasts)

*Figure 1:* **The Immune System at Work**

1. When antibodies are needed, macrophages (M) "hand" antigen (An) to the B-cell. T-helper cells (TH) turn "on" B-cells.

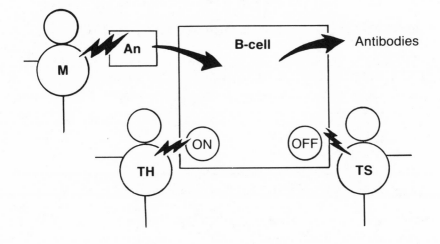

2. When antibodies are no longer needed, T-suppressor cells (TS) turn "off" B-cells.

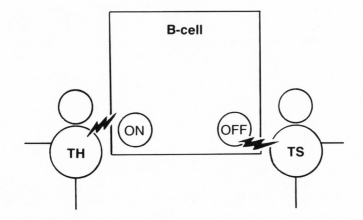

which are waiting to become lymphocytes. Lymphoblasts then enter the circulation through the lymphatic ducts. After maturing, the lymphoblasts move into the tissue below the lining of the intestine, lung, breast, genitourinary tract and female reproductive tract. When they are stimulated by the same antigen which originally started the process they secrete IgA. This process protects the body from foreign substances such as bacteria, viruses, fungi and toxins.

## 6. IMMUNE RESPONSES: COMPONENTS

The immune system responds to foreign substances in two ways: the humoral immune response and the cell-mediated immune response. Each of these responses is triggered by antigens (usually foreign proteins).

### A. *Humoral Response*

The humoral immune response includes the production of antibodies by B-cells and the release of those antibodies into the blood. If you are again exposed to toxins, these antibodies combine with those toxins (antigens) and neutralize them. During an infection, the antibodies coat the surfaces of the microorganisms (bacteria and viruses) and make it easier for the other white blood cells to attack them. This response is your major defense against bacterial infection.

B-cells, T-cells and macrophages are all included in the humoral immune response. B-cells have receptors on their surfaces which link to particular antigens. Think of receptors as being specialized "hooks" which attract and attach to only certain antigens. This attraction and attachment is extremely specialized. It is like a lock and key. When the antigen binds to the B-cell, that cell is stimulated to divide into plasma cells. Plasma cells are the active form of B-cells because they produce antibodies. These plasma cells produce and give off large quantities of antibodies into the blood. Helper T-cells encourage this process and suppressor T-cells discourage it. The number of T-cells which your body produces depends on the physical contact between the T-cells and the macrophages containing the antigen to which the T-cells are responding. If you are exposed to a toxin, the antibodies combine with the antigen (such as a bacterial toxin) and neutralize it; or if you have an infection, the antibodies coat the antigenic surfaces of the microorganisms and make it easier for complement to break them or for the macrophages to digest them.

## B. Cellular Response

The cellular immune response consists of T-cells which have been "sensitized" to foreign antigens. This sensitization occurred sometime in the past when you first came into contact with the harmful foreign substance. When these sensitized T-cells next meet the same foreign antigens, they enlarge, divide and destroy the foreign cells. The cellular immune response is the major defense against infection due to viruses, fungi and a few bacteria.

Effector T-cells are specialized and only recognize what cells and compounds are your own. They do this by recognizing human leukocyte antigens (HLA). (Human leukocyte antigens are called antigens because they are proteins and are capable of causing antibody production. They do not cause your immune system to produce antibodies because your immune system recognizes those antigens as being part of you.) It is the HLA antigens that distinguish "self" from "nonself."[1,2,3]

## 7. WHAT CAN GO WRONG?

The immune system can malfunction in two general ways: in the way it reacts to your own cells and chemical compounds and in the way it reacts to foreign cells and toxins.

Normally, your immune system recognizes your own cells as being part of you and realizes that there is no need to react to them. If your immune system fails to recognize your own cells as "self," then it will sound an alarm and will produce antibodies against your own cells as if they were harmful foreign substances. If this happens, the antibodies which you produce in response to your own cells can destroy your cells or chemical compounds. Not only are your cells and chemical compounds detroyed, but the resulting inflammation and the toxic products produced by the allergic reaction can also be harmful. Physicians describe this reaction to "self" as an autoimmune disease.

How does an otherwise healthy immune system malfunction and attack its own cells or chemical compounds? This malfunction can be brought about in two ways: either through an alteration within the individual's cells or chemical compounds or through an abnormal reaction by the immune system itself.

Cells or chemical compounds can be altered by changes in their chemical structure or when the cells cross react with some foreign substances. An individual's own chemical compounds can be changed if they combine with a chemical or drug. This combination produces a new compound which the body no longer recognizes as self. For example, this alteration can be seen in the changes that occur in red blood cells due to their exposure to certain drugs. The body no longer recognizes these RBCs as being part of itself and attacks and destroys them.

Cross reaction occurs when the antigen of an infectious agent is almost identical to the normal proteins contained within human cells. The antibodies produced against the infectious agent also attack the compounds in the human cell. An example of this cross reaction is seen in rheumatic heart disease following a bacterial (streptococcal) infection.

Autoimmune malfunction also occurs if suppressor T-cells are missing. As you have seen, suppressor T-cells tell B-cells not to produce antibodies. When these T-cells are missing, the B-cells may produce antibodies against our own tissues.

The second way that the immune system can malfunction is in its reaction to foreign substances. This malfunction includes two types of reactions: hypersensitivity and immunologic tolerance. Hypersensitivity occurs when the immune system overreacts to foreign substances. It overreacts according to the same mechanism described in the Humoral Response section (section six of this chapter). This type of reaction may occur when suppressor T-cells are missing or malfunction, or when there is an excess of helper T-cells. Both of these situations result in an increased production of antibodies by the B-cells.

Immunologic tolerance simply means that the immune system "tolerates" foreign substances instead of reacting to them. If this occurs, the individual cannot produce antibodies against a specific antigen (e.g., an infectious agent). A possible reason for this mechanism could be a decreased number of helper T-cells or an increased number of suppressor T-cells, both of which would limit the amount of antibodies produced by the B-cells.

Immunologic tolerance can occur in two ways: by repeated exposure to small doses of antigen (Low Dose Tolerance) or by repeated exposure to large doses of antigen (High Dose Tolerance). An example of Low Dose Tolerance is described by Dr. Truss.[4] Some patients who have a specific fungal infection (Candida albicans) in their intestines fail to react to that infection because, over a period of time, they have been exposed to repeated small doses of Candida toxins. This has resulted in immunologic tolerance to that microorganism. Researchers have found that foreign antigens which are introduced to a fetus before its immune system matures can cause life-long tolerance to the organism which produced the antigen. It is therefore reasonable to assume that a mother with a longstanding untreated Candida infection may allow tolerance of that organism in her offspring.

## 8. EXAMPLES OF IMMUNE MALFUNCTION

The following examples of immune malfunction illustrate the effect which toxins may have on the immune system. The first three examples are of genetic immunodeficiencies which usually result in death during the first two years of life; the fourth example is of acquired immune deficiency (AIDS).

(1) Common Variable Immunodeficiency—is a disease in which the patient has symptoms of a malabsorption of nutrients, is commonly infected by the parasite *Giardia lamblia* and has a high frequency of autoimmune disease. These patients have a normal number of B-cells. However, these B-cells have failed to mature into antibody-producing plasma cells. In addition, the patients may have abnormalities in their T-cells which cause either a lack of T-helper cells or an excess of T-suppressor cells. All of these abnormalities result in decreased antibody production. The purpose of this example is to show that malabsorption of nutrients and opportunistic infections (by parasites or fungi) occur along with immune malfunction.

2) Di George's Syndrome—is a disease in which the thymus gland is missing or extremely small. Because T-cells mature in the thymus, the result of this disease is a deficiency of T-cells. Blood tests indicate that there are either low circulating lymphocytes in the blood or a normal number of lymphocytes but they are all B-cells. This lack of T-cells results in poor defense against fungal and viral infections. This disease is important because a case history[5] discussed in a later chapter relates the T-cell amount with dental fillings.

3) Severe Combined Immunodeficiency (SCID)—is a disease in which individuals have a defect in their T-cells. This defect is due to the lack of an enzyme (adenosine deaminase) in the red blood cells and leukocytes. The enzyme adenosine deaminase is necessary for nucleic acid metabolism (to convert adenosine to inosine). The lack of this enzyme leads to the accumulation of adenosine in the cell which scientists believe causes the cell to die. Because of these events, the individual lacks T-cells, thereby allowing opportunistic organisms such as Candida and viruses to take hold. This disease

demonstrates the importance that a single enzyme has on immune function.

4) Acquired Immune Deficiency Syndrome (AIDS)—is a disease in which the cell-mediated immunity is suppressed because of a deficiency of T-helper cells. In AIDS, the normal T-helper/T-suppressor ratio (usually 2:1) is reversed. The result of this disease is tolerance to most foreign substances including harmful bacteria and viruses.

The responses of our immune system can range from annoying, but trivial, discomforts (hay fever) to potentially fatal diseases (bronchial asthma). The way we react depends on the delicate balance among the various parts of our immune system. I have described some situations which can interfere with this balance. The lack of mature T-cells will result in the absence of cellular immunity. Abnormal T-cells may cause either a decreased production of humoral antibodies if there is a deficiency of helper T-cells, or it may cause an autoimmune disease if there is a lack of suppressor T-cells.[2]

In addition, nutritional deficiencies, toxic chemicals, toxins from yeast (Candida albicans) and environmental molds, or food and inhalant allergic reactions may also cause imbalances within the immune system.[6]

## 9. THE EXPANDED CONCEPT OF ALLERGY

Up to this point, our discussion has centered on what is considered to be the traditional concept of allergy—that a substance enters the body, is recognized as foreign, and the immune system either initiates a non-specific reaction to dispose of the substance or it reacts with a cell-mediated response (T-cells and B-cells) to the substance by producing specific antibodies against that foreign substance. There are some ill-understood mechanisms that occur which do not produce the traditional antibodies in response to environmental substances, but, nevertheless, cause the patient to experience symptoms. These reactions are sometimes referred to as hypersensitivity reactions. Whether these reactions are toxic, hypersensitive or idiosyncratic remains speculative. What is known, is that if the patient avoids these substances, the symptoms go away. Additionally, it is known that if neutralization therapy is undertaken, i.e., injecting a therapeutic dose of the offending substance on a periodic basis, symptoms are reduced. Neutralization therapy, although controversial, is considered to be one of the tools effectively used by those physicians (clinical ecologists) who practice environmental medicine.

# LOOKING BACK

1. The purpose of your immune system is defense. It protects you from bacterial, viral and fungal infections and from toxins. This protection is the result of a finely tuned system of cells and proteins which capture, disable and digest any foreign materials which enter your body.
2. The immune system consists of:
   a. Cells, some of which produce antibodies and some of which attack and digest foreign materials.
   b. Enzymes (complement) which help the actions of antigens and antibodies.
   c. Proteins (antibodies) which attach to or help immobilize foreign materials in order for the macrophages to digest those materials.
3. There are two main immune responses:
   a. The humoral response—an antigen response.
   b. The cellular response—a T-cell and B-cell response.
4. Reactions of the immune system can range from trivial reactions such as hay fever to potentially fatal reactions such as asthma.
5. Malfunctions of the immune system can cause:
   a. Our bodies to fail to recognize our own parts which results in our immune system attacking our own cells.
   b. Our immune system overreacting to normal things in our environment.
   c. Our immune system "tolerating" foreign substances which may be harmful to us.
6. Some of the malfunctions of the immune system are genetic, while others are acquired. Of those acquired malfunctions, nutritional deficiencies, toxic chemicals, toxins from yeast (Candida albicans) and environmental molds, or food and inhalant allergies may contribute to this disease process because of the inflammation and toxic products produced.

## REFERENCES

1. Levin, A. and Dadd, D.: *A Consumer Guide for the Chemically Sensitive*, Levin, A., San Francisco, pp. IX–XVIII, 1982.
2. Ganong, W.: *Review of Medical Physiology*, Lange Medical Publications, Los Altos, California, pp. 414–421, 1983.
3. Robbins, S., Cotran, R. and Kumar, V.: *Pathologic Basis of Disease*, W. B. Saunders, Phila., pp. 158–176, 1984.
4. Truss, C.: *The Missing Diagnosis*, C. Truss, Birmingham, Ala., pp. 21–25, 1983.

5. Eggleston, D.: "Effect of Dental Amalgam and Nickel Alloys of T-lymphocytes: Preliminary Report," *J Pros Dent*, 51(5):617–623, May 1984.

6. Crook, W.: *The Yeast Connection*, Professional Books, Jackson, Tenn., pp. 9–14, 163–166, 1983.

# 4
# MERCURY

LOOKING AHEAD

1. BACKGROUND

2. FORMS OF MERCURY
   A. Mercury Vapor
   B. Mercury Salts
   C. Organic Mercury

3. GENERAL USES OF MERCURY

4. MERCURY EXPOSURE FROM THE ENVIRONMENT

5. MERCURY IN DENTISTRY
   A. Background
   B. Dental Amalgam
   C. The History of Dental Amalgam
   D. Dental Office Exposure

LOOKING BACK

## LOOKING AHEAD

Mercury is one of the heavy metals. It is a silver colored, odorless liquid which evaporates into a colorless, odorless gas at room temperature. Mercury is a poison. It can be found in the ground as mercury ore, and it is used in industry and agriculture. Because of its widespread use, almost everyone is exposed to mercury to some degree in the air they breathe, in the water they drink, and in the food they eat. Unlike other metals (calcium, magnesium, iron, manganese, zinc, copper and chromium) which your body needs for growth, repair, maintenance and defense, mercury has not been found to be beneficial to your health.

In addition to the mercury which is found in air, food and water, you are exposed to mercury every time you go to the dental office. Mercury has been used in dentistry for over 150 years. Its use was very crude at first, but developments in technology and research have improved the quality and reliability of the materials used in dental amalgam fillings. In this chapter I will discuss the forms of mercury, its use, and your potential exposure to mercury. Since most people have dental fillings containing mercury, I will also discuss the history and use of mercury in dentistry. Both scientists and the general public are concerned about whether this dental exposure is harmful to the health of dentists, dental staff and patients. Your exposure to dental mercury is only one part of your total mercury exposure.

## 1. BACKGROUND

Mercury has fascinated man since its discovery about 5,000 years ago. Its silvery appearance gave it its nickname "quicksilver." Because of its silvery appearance, scientists made futile attempts to convert it into gold.

Only a few parts of the world contain natural deposits of mercury ore. In the United States, deposits can be found in Humboldt County, Nevada and Sonoma County, California. In these deposits mercury is found as a metal and as a salt.[1] Because of its use and abuse in industry and agriculture, mercury also occurs in the environment as pollution. As a consequence, mercury is sometimes found in our food and water (drinking water, processed foods and beverages). The concentration of mercury in the air ranges from 1.0 $ng/m^3$ over oceans to tens of thousands of $ng/m^3$ near mercury ore deposits and areas of volcanic activity.

Scientists have estimated the daily human consumption of mercury to be:[2]

1.  air = less than 60 ng/24 hour period (0.60 ug)
2.  water = less than 2 ng/day (0.002 ug)
3.  food = 5,000 to 10,000 ng/day (5 to 10 ug)

NOTE: Since you need to know scientific notation to understand the concentrations of toxins in the air or in a liquid such as blood or urine, I want to give you a brief description of the terms used by scientists. Scientists use the metric system to measure things. The measurement terms are:

1.  The gram  (g) is a unit of weight.
    (1 ounce = 28.3g)
2.  The liter  (l) is a unit of capacity.
    (1.06 quart = 1l)
3.  The meter (m) is a unit of length.
    (39.37 inches = 1m)

In order to express small quantities in standard numbers, scientists break down these terms further:

1.  centi = 1/100th (one hundredth)
2.  milli = 1/1000th (one thousandth)
3.  micro = 1/1,000,000th (one millionth)
4.  nano = 1/1,000,000,000th (one billionth)

Therefore, a microgram (ug) is one millionth of a gram, a nanogram (ng) is one billionth of a gram and a milliliter (ml) is one thousandth of a liter. The term $m^3$ is used to express a cubic meter; that is, a cube measuring a meter on all sides. In this book, this term refers to the amount of air that can be contained in a cube having the measurement of one meter on all sides.

## 2. FORMS OF MERCURY

There are three forms of mercury: the metal (mercury), mercury salt and organic mercurials. In its metallic form, mercury is not considered toxic; but mercury vapor, the gaseous form of mercury, is toxic. These toxic forms of mercury are classified in descending order of toxicity (beginning with the most toxic):[3]

Methyl mercury > mercury vapor > inorganic salts

## A. Mercury Vapor

The metal, mercury, is a liquid at room temperature. As a liquid, some of its atoms evaporate to form a gas which is called mercury vapor. You are familiar with evaporation, because humidity results from water becoming a gas (water vapor). Mercury vapor is considered to be the most dangerous form of mercury because it is a colorless, odorless gas.[4] Because it is colorless and odorless you may not be aware that you are being exposed to mercury. Because of this, it is difficult for you to protect yourself from this type of mercury exposure.

Mercury vapor can cause either acute or chronic toxicity and may also cause an allergic reaction.[5]

## B. Mercury Salts

Mercury salts are a combination of mercury and other chemical elements. For example, mercurous chloride (calomel) is an ingredient in skin cream. Years ago, mercuric nitrate was used in the felt hat industry. It caused neurological and behavioral changes among the workers in that industry. You may recall the "Mad Hatter" character in Lewis Carroll's *Alice in Wonderland* who characterized this type of behavior.[6] Mercuric chloride, once used in antiseptics, was often used by suicide victims. Today, mercury is still used in industry. Because it is discarded in lakes and streams, it continues to be a source of pollution and therefore a potential contaminant in the food chain.

## C. Organic Mercury—Methyl Mercury

Organic mercurials (alkyl mercury compounds) consist of mercury in combination with a carbon-containing compound (organic compound). Methyl mercury is the most commonly known in this class of chemical compounds. An individual who is exposed to methyl mercury has a greater chance for a toxic reaction since methyl mercury is 100 to 1,000 times as toxic as mercury vapor. Methyl mercury is considered to be the most toxic form of mercury because it causes permanent damage. An example of methyl mercury toxicity was found during the 1970s in the Minamata Bay disaster (Japan) where 121 people were poisoned and 46 died because they ate fish which had a high concentration of methyl mercury. These fish had a diet of microorganisms which biotransformed the metallic mercury in the water into methyl mercury. Some of the symptoms associated with Minamata victims included disturbances in intelligence, body growth, speech and limb formation. Children had a high incidence of mental retardation and a 7 percent mortality rate.[6,7]

Alkyl mercury compounds used as fungicides in agriculture caused another mercury catastrophe. In this case, people in Iraq (1972) ate wheat and barley seeds which were prepared for planting by treating them with alkyl mercury. Eating the treated seeds resulted in neurological damage (including delayed mental, speech and motor development) to several thousand people and death to several hundred people.

Even though I have discussed mercury in three categories, in reality, it is difficult to separate the forms of mercury. When we discuss a living organism, the distinctions are not clear cut because mercury may change forms once it is in the body. For example, when mercury vapor is inhaled and enters the blood stream, it is oxidized to mercuric ions. Therefore, laboratory tests do not always tell us what form of mercury an individual was exposed to.

## 3. USES OF MERCURY

Mercury is used in drugs, medicines, industry and dentistry. In the past, mercury was an ingredient in drugs such as diuretics, antiseptics, skin ointments and laxatives; today, mercury has been replaced by less toxic and more effective ingredients. This change has reduced the occurrence of mercury poisoning.[6] The greatest industrial use of mercury is in electrochemistry. Mercury is used in its metallic form in the electrolysis of brine, in thermometers, in mercury street lights and in sun lamps. The salt form of mercury is used in some drugs, fungicides, insecticides, paint pigments and as a detonator in explosive caps.

Mercury poisoning has recently become a problem because of environmental pollution. The concentration of mercury in the air, soil and water has increased because of its use in industry and agriculture. This pollution has led to both wildlife and human mercury poisoning. These incidents of mercury poisoning have often been misdiagnosed because of the gradual onset and vagueness of the symptoms and the practicing physician's unfamiliarity with the disease.[6]

## 4. MERCURY EXPOSURE FROM THE ENVIRONMENT

As you have seen, you can be exposed to mercury from the pollution in air, from the contamination in water and from foods, especially seafood, which may contain methyl mercury. Cosmetics (skin creams and hair dyes) and medications (mercurochrome, merthiolate, ointments and lotions) which contain mercury compounds are another source of exposure. In addition, many items which you may use in your home (paints, laundry aids, fungicides and batteries) contain mercury.

Occupational exposure to mercury can occur among workers who are involved in the manufacture of thermometers, barometers, embalming fluids, insecticides, explosive devices and other products containing mercury.

Finally, you can be exposed to mercury in the dental office. This exposure occurs when the dentist removes or places an amalgam filling in your mouth. There is now scientific evidence which suggests that mercury is also given off by the amalgam fillings in your mouth during chewing and during the normal corrosion process of the filling.[25–38]

## 5. MERCURY IN DENTISTRY

### A. Background

Many metals are used in dentistry; mercury is one of these metals. Other metals include aluminum, beryllium, cadmium, calcium, chromium, cobalt, copper, gold, iron, mercury, nickel, palladium, platinum, silver, titanium, tin, vanadium and zinc (see Table 1).[8] Dentists use these metals for:

a. dental fillings
b. prosthetic devices, such as partial dentures which require a metal base
c. bridgework, which requires a metal base to span across the space left by a missing tooth
d. single crowns (caps), which use a metal base
e. implants, which are used if bone was lost on the lower jaw
f. orthodontic treatment appliances (braces)

Mercury is used in combination with other metals in the fabrication of fillings. Those fillings which are made from mercury in combination with other metals are called *dental amalgams*.

Table 1 summarizes the metals that are used in dentistry, their potential to be toxic and their potential to cause allergy. Of the metals listed, there has been toxicity reported in the scientific literature in the non-dental use of beryllium, chromium, mercury and nickel. This toxicity has been caused by dust created in connec-

## Table 1: METALS USED IN DENTISTRY

| Metal | Dental Use | Reported Non-Dental Toxicity | Non-Dental Form | Reported Dental Toxicity | Reported Dental Allergy |
|---|---|---|---|---|---|
| 1. Aluminum | temp. crowns | | | no | |
| 2. Beryllium | prosthetics | yes | occup. dust | no | |
| 3. Calcium | therapeutics | | | no | |
| 4. Chromium | prosthetics | yes | occup. dust | no | yes |
| 5. Cobalt | prosthetics | | | no | yes |
| 6. Copper | restorations | | | | |
| 7. Gold | rest./prosth. | | | no | yes |
| 8. Iron | ortho. appl. | | | no | |
| 9. Mercury | restorations | yes | mercury vapor, inorg. mercury | yes | yes |
| 10. Nickel | prosthetics | yes | org. mercury, occup. dust | yes | yes |
| 11. Palladium | prosthetics | | | | yes |
| 12. Platinum | prosthetics | | | | yes |
| 13. Silver | restorations | | | | yes |
| 14. Titanium | prosthetics | | | | |
| 15. Tin | restorations | | | | |
| 16. Vanadium | prosthetics | | | | |
| 17. Zinc | restorations | | | | |

| Metal | Reported Percent Affected | Allergy Site | Oral Site | Allergy Test |
|---|---|---|---|---|
| 1. Aluminum | | | | |
| 2. Beryllium | | | | |
| 3. Calcium | | | | |
| 4. Chromium | | | | |
| 5. Cobalt | 1% | local | yes | patch |
| 6. Copper | | local | | |
| 7. Gold | | | | |
| 8. Iron | | | | |
| 9. Mercury | <1% | local/systemic | | patch |
| 10. Nickel | female = 10% male = <1% | local/systemic | yes | patch |
| 11. Palladium | | | | |
| 12. Platinum | | | | |
| 13. Silver | | | | |
| 14. Titanium | | | | |
| 15. Tin | | | | |
| 16. Vanadium | | | | |
| 17. Zinc | | | | |

tion with the individual's occupation. Both toxicity and allergy have been reported when mercury and nickel were used in dental restorations. Dental allergy has been noted with the use of chromium, cobalt, gold, mercury, nickel, palladium, platinum, and silver. An interesting but unexplained statistic is that nickel allergy affects more than 10 times the number of women than it does men. Of the metals listed, only chromium and nickel have produced signs of allergy or toxicity in the mouth. Some researchers have suggested that some cases of gingivitis are an oral manifestation of mercury allergy. Allergy to an individual metal is usually confirmed through patch testing.

### B. Dental Amalgam

In order for you to understand dental amalgam, you must be familiar with several terms. The first term is "alloy," which is simply a combination of two or more metals. In dentistry, silver, tin, and copper make up the "dental alloy." When we add mercury to that dental alloy it forms an amalgam. An "amalgam" is the combination of mercury with one or more other metals. Therefore, a combination of mercury with the dental alloy containing silver, tin, copper, and sometimes zinc forms a brand-new alloy called "dental amalgam." These metallic compounds are held together by intermetallic bonding which results in a solid solution of metals. Intermetallic bonding can be described as "tight hand holding." Each metal holds on to the other metals because of their strong positive and negative charges. In the dental amalgam, the final proportion of mercury to dental alloy is 1:1 (50 percent alloy to 50 percent mercury by weight). In mixing dental amalgam, the dentist and his staff are careful to insure that there is no excess mercury in your filling. Too much mercury leads to excessive expansion and loss of strength in the filling. The result of this expansion and loss of strength is your having to replace your fillings more often.[9]

### C. History of Dental Amalgam

France was the first country to use dental amalgam (1826) followed by the United States several years later (1833). Early amalgam, probably made by mixing mercury with the filings of silver coins, was an inferior product by present day standards. Amalgam research and improvements were made during the next several decades. In 1929 the American Dental Association (ADA) adopted Specification #1 for amalgam. This specification was the result of studies conducted at the National Bureau of Standards. More recent research and development by dental manufacturing companies, scientists and clinicians have further improved the amalgam alloy. Today, the metals used in amalgam are refined and proportioned. Dentists depend on state-of-the-art technology to produce a consistent and reliable product: your amalgam filling.[9]

As you know, the alloy used to make dental amalgam contains silver, tin, copper and sometimes zinc. The acceptable range of measurement for these metals are as follows:

## PERCENTAGE BY WEIGHT

| Alloy | ADA Spec. #1 | Typical Alloy | Range |
|-------|--------------|---------------|-------|
| silver | 65 (min) | 69.0 | 65–74 |
| tin | 29 (max) | 27.0 | 24–29 |
| copper | 6 (max) | 3.0 | 0–6 |
| zinc | 2 (max) | 1.0 | 0–2 |

Each of the ingredients in the dental amalgam has a specific function. The purpose for using silver in dental amalgam is for strength and fast setting (hardening). Tin helps in amalgamation (mixing of mercury with the dental alloy) and it aids in reducing expansion. Copper improves the strength, hardness and setting of the amalgam. Zinc is used by the manufacturers during the production of the alloy.[9,10]

### D. Dental Office Exposure

In the dental office, dentists and dental staff are exposed to mercury because of poor mercury hygiene and from the mercury vapor which is unavoidably produced during the restorative process (during the process of removing, mixing and placing an amalgam filling).[11–14,16] Poor mercury hygiene also occurs when mercury is not carefully handled or when it is improperly stored. Because mercury is a liquid, careless handling can result in spillage. If spilled, mercury seeps into cracks and crevices of carpeting, wood flooring and dental equipment; it will continually evaporate and form mercury vapor which will contaminate the air over a long period of time. Because it is colorless and odorless, detection and clean-up of spilled mercury is very difficult. Detection of spilled mercury can only be accomplished by special mercury detection instruments. Dentists and the dental staff must first be aware that mercury can be poisonous and then must be motivated to monitor the mercury level in the office. Government agencies have established acceptable levels of mercury in the workplace. Although the amount of mercury vapor in the dental office may be below this acceptable level (TLV), it is, nonetheless, an exposure to mercury. (TLV—The Threshold Limit Value for mercury vapor by the United States Standards is 50 ug/m$^3$ over a series of five daily exposure periods of eight hours each during a one week interval. The TLV for the USSR is 10 ug/m$^3$.)[12]

Dental staff can be exposed to mercury either by direct contact with metallic mercury, by handling mercury compounds or by inhaling mercury vapors. Although contaminated office spaces will predominately affect the dental staff, patients will also be exposed to the mercury in the air during their dental visit.

If the building where the dental office is located contains other offices, contaminated air can be carried into those other offices. This occurs when the building has central hot air heating and/or central air conditioning. An example of this situation is the typical shopping mall dental practice. In a mall dental practice, the office is usually located within a department store or complex of stores with the waiting room/reception area opened to the general corridor space. The heating and cooling is provided either through a central or sectionalized system. Therefore, the same air is circulated to all stores and offices that are contained within the system.[17]

Patients are also exposed to mercury during the removal of an old amalgam filling and during the placement of a new amalgam filling. The specific steps occurring within the dental office include:

1. Removal of the old amalgam filling, if any
2. Mixing of the new amalgam filling
3. Placement of the new amalgam filling
4. Carving and adjustment of the new amalgam filling

After the amalgam filling is placed in your tooth, you can still be exposed to mercury through the vaporization of mercury from your fillings. This vaporization results from the mechanical wear of the filling and from corrosion. Mechanical wear occurs whenever you chew, grind your teeth or brush your teeth. Corrosion is the normal and gradual wearing away of the filling because of chemical action. In short, this chemical action occurs because the metal in the amalgam reacts with the chemicals in your mouth. Mechanical wear and corrosion occurs with both new fillings and old fillings. The mercury vapor given off by wear and corrosion can penetrate into the dental tubules in your teeth and into the soft tissue (gums) adjacent to the amalgam filling.[18–27,29–31,33,36–38]

# LOOKING BACK

1. Mercury exists in air, food and water.
2. The metal, mercury, has been known to man for about 5,000 years.
3. Mercury compounds occur naturally in the ground and in pollutants in the atmosphere and in the food chain.
4. Metallic mercury is present in dental amalgam fillings.
5. Mercury and its compounds are used as drugs, in industry, and in agriculture.
6. The forms of mercury are:
   a. Metallic mercury (mercury vapor)—the most dangerous.
   b. Mercury salts—very toxic.
   c. Organic mercury (methyl mercury)—the most toxic.
7. Dentistry uses products from all sources: metals, minerals, petrochemicals, inorganic chemicals, sea agar, resins, oils and waxes.[39]
8. Mercury is only one metal used in dentistry, but it is not the only metal of allergic or toxic concern.
9. Metals used in dentistry which are also of great allergic concern are chromium, cobalt, gold, nickel, palladium, platinum, and silver.
10. Dental amalgam (mercury, silver, tin, copper, and sometimes zinc) has been used in dentistry for approximately 150 years.
11. Dentists and dental staff are exposed to mercury in the office through careless handling, improper storage and the mercury unavoidably given off during the fabrication of an amalgam filling.
12. Patients are exposed to mercury from their amalgam fillings.

## REFERENCES

1. Hutchinson, E.: *Chemistry: The Elements and Their Reactions*, W.B. Saunders Co., Philadelphia, 1964.
2. Stokinger, H.: *Patty's Industrial Hygiene and Technology: Metals Section*, 3rd edition, John Wiley and Sons, New York, p. 1779.
3. "Safety of Dental Amalgam," Council on Dental Materials, Instruments and Equipment and Council of Dental Therapeutics, *JADA*, vol. 106, April, 1983.
4. Kawahara, H., Nakamura, H., Yamagami, A., and Nakanishi, T.: "Cellular Responses to Dental Amalgam in Vitro," *J Dent Res*, 54(2):394–401, March-April, 1975.
5. Cooley, R. and Young, J.: "Detection and Diagnosis of Bioincompatibility of Mercury," *CDA Journal*, 12(1):36–43, October 1984.
6. Gilman, A., Goodman, L. and Gilman, A.: *The Pharmacological Basis of Therapeutics*, Macmillan Pub. Co., New York, 1980.

7. Bakir, F., Al-Khalidi, A., Clarkson, T. and Greenwald, R.: "Classical Observation on Treatment of Alkylmercury Poisoning in Hospital Patients," Bull. WHO 53(supp):87–92, 1976.

8. "Workshop: Biocompatibility of Metals in Dentistry," National Institute of Dental Research, *JADA*, 109:469–471, September 1984.

9. Craig, R. and Peyton, F. (editors): *Restorative Dental Materials*, C.V. Mosby Co., 5th edition, pp. 123–129; 169–170, St. Louis, 1975.

10. O'Brien, W. and Ryge, G.: *An Outline of Dental Materials*, W. B. Saunders Co., Philadelphia, pp. 210–211, 1978.

11. "Objections to the Use of Amalgam for Filling Teeth," (Berlin Letter), *J Amer Med Assoc*, 90:1056–1057, March 1928.

12. Berlin, M., Clarkson, T., Friberg, L., Gage, L., Goldwater, L., Jernelov, A., Kazantzis, G., Magos, L., Nordberg, G., Radford, E., Ramel, C., Skerfving, S., Smith, R., Suzuki, T., Swensson, A., Tejning, S., Trukart, R. and Vostol, J.: "Report of an International Committee: Maximum Allowable Concentrations of Mercury Compounds," *Arch Environ Health*, 19:891–905, December 1969.

13. Abraham, J., Svare, C. and Frank, C.: "The Effects of Dental Amalgam Restorations on Blood Mercury Levels," *J Dent Res*, 63(1):71–73, 1984.

14. Gaul, L.: "Immunity of the Oral Mucosa in Epidermal Sensitization to Mercury," *Arch Dermat*, 93(1):45–46, January 1966.

15. Leirskar, J.: "On the Mechanisms of Cytotoxicity of Silver and Copper Amalgams in a Cell System," *Scand J Dent Res*, 82(1):74–81, 1974.

16. Lintz, W.: "Prevention and Cure of Occupational Diseases of the Dentist," *J Amer Dent Assoc*, 22(12):2071–2081, December 1935.

17. Zamm, A. and Gannon, R.: *Why Your House May Endanger Your Health*, Simon and Schuster, New York, pp. 46– 60, 109–110, 135–167, 1980.

18. Freden, H., Hellden, L. and Milledig, P.: "Mercury Content in Gingival Tissues Adjacent to Amalgam Fillings," *Odonto Revy*, 25(2):207–210, 1974.

19. Rupp, N, and Paffenbarger, J.: "Significance to Health of Mercury Used in Dental Practice: A Review," *J Amer Dent Assoc*, 82(6):1401–1407, June 1971.

20. "Media Message Misleads," *ADA News* (Chicago), November 21, 1983.

21. "Experts to Review Safety of Metals in Dentistry," ADA News (Chicago), December 1983.

22. "Dentists, Staff Members Healthy, Despite Daily Contact with Mercury," *ADA News* (Chicago), December 1983.

23. "Criteria for a Recommended Standard: Occupational Exposure to Inorganic Mercury" National Institute of Occupational Safety and Health, (Public Health Service, U.S. Dept. of HEW, 1973).

24. Bauer, J. and First, H.: "The Toxicity of Mercury in Dental Amalgam," *J Calif Dent Assoc*, 10:47–61, June 1982.

25. Utt, H.: "Mercury Breath . . . How much is too much?" *CDA Journal*, 12(2):41–45, February 1984.

26. Cooley, R. and Young, J.: "Detection and Diagnosis of Bioincompatibility of Mercury," *CDA Journal*, 12(10):36–43, October 1984.
27. Anusavice, K., Soderholm, K., Mohammed, H, and Shen, C.: "Consequences of Mercury Exposure in Dentistry: A Review of the Literature," *Fla Dent J*, 54(4):17–19, Winter 1983.
28. Leirskar, J.: "On the Mechanisms of Cytotoxicity of Silver and Copper Amalgams in a Cell System," *Scand J Dent Res*, 82(1):74–81, 1974.
29. Frykholm, K.: "On Mercury from Dental Amalgam, Its Toxic and Allergic Effects and some Comments on Occupational Hygiene," *Acata Odont Scand*, 15(suppl 22):1–108, 1957.
30. Svare, C., Frank, C. and Chan, K.: "Quantative Measure of Mercury Vapor Emission from Setting Dental Amalgam," *J Dent Res*, 52:740–743, July-Aug, 1973.
31. Svare, C.: "Dental Amalgam Related Mercury Vapor Exposure," *CDA Journal*, 17(10):54–58, October, 1948.
32. Chan, K. and Svare, C.: "Mercury Vapor Emission from Dental Amalgam," *J Dent Res*, pp. 555–559, March-April 1972.
33. Svare, C., Peterson, L., Reinhardt, J., Frank, C. and Boyer, D.: "Dental Amalgam: A Potential Source of Mercury Vapor Exposure," *J of Dent Res*, 59 (Special Issue A):391, Abstract #293, March 1980.
34. Svare, C., Peterson, L., Reinhardt, J., Boyer, D., Frank, C., Gay, D. and Cox, R.: "The Effects of Dental Amalgams on Mercury Levels in Expired Air," *J Dent Res*, 60(9):1668–1671, September, 1981.
35. Hursh, J. Clarkson, T., Cherian, M., Vostal, J. and Vander Malie, R.: "Clearance of Mercury Vapor Inhaled by Human Subjects," *Arch Environ Health*, 31:302–309, 1976.
36. Moller, B.: "Reactions of Human Dental Pulp to Silver Amalgam Restorations, Mercury Determination in Dental Pulps by Flameless Atomic Absorption Spectrophotometry," *Swed Dent J*, 2:93–97, 1978.
37. Holland, G. and Asgar, K.: "Some Effects on the Phases of Amalgam Induced by Corrosion," *J Dent Res*, 53:1245–1254, 1974.
38. Pleva, J.: "Mercury Poisoning From Dental Amalgam," *Orthomolecular Psychiatry*, 12(3):184–193, 1983.
39. Fasciana, G.: *Dental Materials: An Outline for the Allergic and Chemically Sensitive Patient*, Fasciana, G. 106 Nassau Drive, Springfield, Mass., 1983.

# 5
# THE
# CONTROVERSY

# LOOKING AHEAD

Dentists have always been able to choose from a large selection of dental materials. Most of these materials were and still are the "standard" in dentistry. These standard materials have been considered to be effective, predictable and safe; they are the materials that every dentist learns to use in dental school. During the last fifteen years, the number of dental materials on the market has skyrocketed. Many of these materials are made from petrochemicals: impression materials, composite fillings, denture base materials, cements, etc.

Practicing dentists today have a wide choice of dental materials. How do dentists choose from these materials? They will select materials with which they feel most comfortable because they are able to work with the material and it produces the results they desire. How do dentists become comfortable with the material? First, they probably prefer those materials which they were taught to use in dental school. However, because of the new dental materials available combined with dentists' desire for perfection, dentists are always trying to improve both the materials and procedures used in their offices. Because the average dentist has a small practice with a limited number of patients, evaluation of the performance of the dental materials on these patients is limited. To evaluate the safety of the dental materials, your dentist must depend on the opinions of scientists and manufacturers who develop and test these dental materials.

In general, the dental profession accepts a wide variety of dental procedures and dental materials as long as these materials and procedures have been demonstrated to be safe. When you visit your dentist for a check-up, your dentist evaluates your dental needs and recommends treatment. Your dentist's recommendation is based on experience, your specific needs and the materials which your dentist feels will be long lasting and cost-effective. Amalgam fillings are usually recommended whenever a strong and durable filling is required. Amalgam is a filling material which your dentist has been trained to use, is comfortable with, is considered safe by the American Dental Association and is cost-effective.

As you have seen, the safety of dental amalgam has been controversial since its introduction to the dental profession. Scientists have not been able to agree on whether the mercury in dental amalgam is toxic. This chapter discusses the controversy surrounding dental mercury. Since dentists and patients must depend on the opinions and conclusions of researchers and scientists concerning the safety of dental mercury, I have included a section describing how scientific research is selected for publication.

## 1. BACKGROUND

The debate concerning the safety of dental mercury is in the forefront of scientific literature. The controversy about dental mercury has centered around two schools of thought: the pro-mercury group and the anti-mercury group. The pro-mercury group maintains that mercury is safe and that dental mercury causes no adverse effects except in only the "most sensitive individuals" which includes less than 1 percent of the population. The American Dental Association is the main proponent of this position.

The opposing group in the debate (the anti-mercury group) maintains that mercury is a health hazard which contributes to or causes a range of diseases including those which affect the nervous system, circulatory system, connective tissues and the immune system. The major advocates of this position include Hal Huggins, D.D.S. and Sam Ziff.

As with most controversies, each group advances strong arguments by using clinical experience and published research to strengthen their claim. They also minimize or refute opposing conclusions or clinical experiences of researchers and clinicians.

Our challenge is to sift through the clinical claims, published case histories and published research concerning mercury and health. Then we must determine which view appears to be more valid. Given our present knowledge and state of the art technology, there may not be a definitive right or wrong answer which applies to everyone. We will evaluate the arguments, we will evaluate the scientific literature and we will evaluate the alternative filling materials. Then you must apply your philosophy of health to this evaluation and make your decision as to whether dental mercury is harmful to your health.

## 2. PUBLICATIONS

We all have a tendency to believe what we read. Scientific articles generally have more credibility. Most people believe that scientific theories can either be proved or disproved, and, therefore, scientific beliefs are either right or wrong. In addition, credibility depends on the credentials of the author and the reputation of the magazine or journal. For instance, on the subject of nutrition, which would you believe: *The Star* or the *New England Journal of Medicine?* Let's make it a little bit more difficult! Would you believe the *New England Journal of Medicine* or a smaller, not as well known, medical journal? The fact is, that it is often easy to distinguish credibility between a scientific publication and non-scientific publication concerning the topic of health. More difficult is distinguishing the credibility among reputable, but less well known, scientific journals. This is not to imply that the lesser-known scientific journal contains information which is less credible than the information contained in the most popular journals; but, people may more readily accept the conclusions presented in the more popular journals.

As you can see from this discussion, not everything that you read should carry the same weight. You must be an alert, discriminating reader! There are several levels at which data can be presented. The first and the most objective level is the reporting of scientific research published in medical journals and science journals. This information is the most objective because the research must follow certain procedures known as the scientific method. This method includes the researcher defining a problem, collecting data through observation and experiment and formulating and testing a hypothesis.

The second level of reporting is, for example, a literature review. In a literature review, many published research articles are compiled by the literature review author. The literature review author makes conclusions based on these reports, each of which may have come to a slightly different conclusion. The final conclusions which the literature review author synthesizes from these published articles allow for greater subjectivity.

When book authors quote or refer to a research publication, they see the data from their own perspective. Therefore, a book which quotes research is more subjective than scientific findings published in a journal because there is a range of interpretation that is possible depending on the author's purpose and personal beliefs. Therefore, the further the author is from the research, the greater the subjectivity.

The types of reports published in scientific journals include case histories, literature reviews and scientific research studies. The information contained in these publications was essential in writing this book. I want to share with you the criteria that most scientific journals use to judge manuscripts which are submitted for publication. These criteria include:

1) The subject matter of the articles which the journal publishes,
2) The methods used by the author to do the research,
3) The technical or experimental design of the research,
4) The references used by the author,
5) The illustrations and tables used to present data,
6) The soundness of the author's conclusions and
7) The existence of a "double-blind" control.

What steps are involved in having an article published in a scientific journal? The process of publication involves submitting a manuscript to the scientific journal. The author's manuscript is then sent to three reviewers for an unbiased critical evaluation. The author is not identified in order to be anonymous to the reviewers. These reviewers are usually recognized authorities on the subject matter discussed in the manuscript. The decision made by the reviewers determines whether the submitted manuscript will be published in that scientific journal.

Some of the reasons journals have given for rejecting a manuscript include:

1) The subject matter of the manuscript is not suitable for that particular publication,
2) The organization, information, references, objectivity or writing ability of the author fall short of the standards set by the publication,
3) The design of experimental or technical data is flawed and
4) The data does not support the conclusion.

There is an additional factor involved in the rejection of a manuscript. This factor is the potential bias of the reviewer. Although the manuscripts are submitted to each reviewer for an unbiased evaluation, the objectivity of the review can be compromised in at least two ways: if the reviewer is not open-minded or feels that his or her published conclusions are being threatened by a new hypothesis or an opposing conclusion. These biases, however unlikely, need to be recognized as a factor for the rejection of a manuscript for publication.

As you can see, publication of scientific articles is not an automatic process. The purpose for this strict review process is to maintain the high standards necessary to maintain credibility and dependability of scientific literature. If all authors had their articles published without regard to their scientific truth, the scientific community could no longer rely on any published information. Even though there are times when a valuable piece of research or enlightening case history is not published, on balance, the system works.

In conclusion, there are some valuable articles which were never accepted for publication; there are some articles which have been published because they add support to the present beliefs of the scientific community. You must be aware that the scientific literature may not contain all relevant information and that scientific beliefs are not written in stone, but they change and grow as does every body of knowledge.[1]

## LOOKING BACK

1. Mercury has been used in dentistry for about 150 years.
2. There have been periods in which dentists and/or researchers have questioned the safety of the mercury used in dental amalgam fillings.
3. The present controversy about dental mercury has been predominantly between two groups.
4. The pro-mercury group believes that mercury in dental fillings is safe; the anti-mercury group believes that the mercury in dental fillings is toxic and causes or contributes to a wide variety of diseases.
5. Both groups cite scientific literature to support their respective positions.
6. The shortcoming of scientific literature is that it may not be a complete accounting of all information available.

### REFERENCES

1. Compiled from the "information for authors" section of the following journals: *Journal of the American Dental Association, Journal of the Canadian Dental Association, Clinical Ecology, Journal of Prosthetic Dentistry*, and the *Journal of the Academy of General Dentistry*.

# 6
# THE
# PRO-MERCURY
# POSITION

LOOKING AHEAD

1. BACKGROUND

2. PRO-MERCURY POSITION

3. QUICK REFERENCE OUTLINE (PRO-MERCURY)

4. EVALUATION

LOOKING BACK

# LOOKING AHEAD

Of the 126,985 licensed dentists in the United States, 119,177 (94 percent) are members of the American Dental Association (ADA).[1] The ADA has always been regarded as *the* authority on dental procedures, dental therapeutics, dental materials, instruments and equipment; the ADA continues to hold this positon of authority today. This chapter discusses the ADA (pro-mercury) position on the safety of dental amalgam.

## 1. BACKGROUND

The pro-mercury group admists that dentists, dental staff and patients are exposed to mercury vapor during the removal of, the mixing of and the placement of amalgam fillings (during the restorative process), but maintains that this exposure is within acceptable levels and well below the Threshold Limit Value (TLV) recommended by the Occupational Safety and Health Administration (OSHA). The TLV for mercury in the United States is 50 ug/m$^3$ based on a time-weighed average during an 8 hour workday for a consecutive 5 day work period. (See Appendix II for information on government standards.)

The American Dental Association (ADA) has stated that:

> ". . . the most important point to be made about dental use of mercury is that the dentist and dental personnel, not the patient, are the people who would be most at risk to potential mercury hazards"[2] and that "dental professionals are a generally healthy group of individuals who show no ill effects from their contact with mercury."[3]

The ADA further acknowledges:

> ". . . that in extremely rare cases patients may develop a hypersensitivity or allergy from contact with mercury, a condition that usually turns up as skin rash and is similar to other common allergies. The fact that a very small percentage of the population is hypersensitive to mercury should not be cause for alarm."[4]

An extensive 1982 literature review by Bauer[5] is quoted by the ADA to support its claim of dental amalgam safety. Bauer concluded that: ". . . [our review] indicates that the use of mercury in dental amalgam is relatively safe. The potential for mercury poisoning exists; however, it is negligible."

## 2. PRO-MERCURY POSITION[2-4,6-11]

I have organized the pro-mercury position into seven major categories. The topics I will discuss include:

(1) Sources of Mercury Exposure in the Dental Office
(2) Symptoms and Injuries Resulting from High Doses and/or Chronic Mercury Exposure
(3) Symptoms or Signs Resulting from Allergic Reactions
(4) Biological Responses to Mercury Exposure
(5) Mercury Testing Service Available for Dental Staff
(6) The Health of Dental Staff
(7) ADA Recommendations for the Replacement of Amalgam Fillings

(1) *Sources of Mercury Exposure in the Dental Office*—The ADA asserts that dentists and dental staff can be exposed to mercury in two ways: direct contact and inhalation. Exposure to mercury from direct contact (handling) may occur during the restorative process by dental staff touching the mercury or amalgam mixture. The second possible manner of mercury exposure is the inhalation of mercury vapors which are given off during the restorative process or mercury vapors produced as a result of poor mercury hygiene. Poor mercury hygiene is the careless handling of metallic mercury or the improper storage of excess amalgam left over from fillings. Either of these activities produces mercury vapor which contaminates the office air.

(2) *Symptoms and Injuries Resulting from High Doses and/or Chronic Mercury Exposure*—The main symptoms which the ADA identifies as resulting from high doses or chronic mercury exposure include: neurological (tremor, depression, irritability, moodiness, nervous excitability and headache), gastrointestinal (ulceration of the oral mucosa, loss of appetite, nausea and diarrhea), fatigue, swollen glands and tongue, insomnia, dark pigmentation of the gums, and loosening of teeth.

(3) *Symptoms or Signs Resulting from Allergic Reactions*—The two symptoms or signs indicated by the ADA as resulting from an allergic reaction to mercury are localized dermatitis (inflammation of the skin) and generalized erythema (inflammatory redness of the skin).

(4) *Biological Responses to Mercury Exposure*—The ADA recognizes that exposure to mercury results in the accumulation of mer-

cury in the kidney, liver, brain and heart muscle. The central nervous system (CNS) is especially sensitive to mercury because of its high lipid (fat) content and its slow elimination of mercury. Mercury acts on the nervous system by "blocking the metabolism" of the individual nerve cell.

(5) *Mercury Testing Service Available for Dental Staff*—The ADA provides mercury testing for dentists and dental staff. Between January, 1982 and November, 1983, 776 dentists and their staff were tested. The results of this testing were that dental personnel had an average urine mercury of 14.6 ug/l compared with 3.0 ug/l for the general population.

(6) *Health of Dental Staff*—The ADA quotes a study by Shapiro which indicated that of 298 dentists studied, 23 had tissue mercury levels above 20 ug/g. Thirty percent of the 23 dentists with high tissue mercury had polyneuropathies (diseases of peripheral nerves) which resulted in visual impairment.[12]

(7) *Recommendations for the Replacement of Amalgam Fillings*— The ADA maintains that a sound healthy tooth will suffer structural loss when a filling is removed. This structural loss may result in the need for root canal treatment or the loss of the tooth. The alternatives to amalgam are gold, which would not likely be covered by the patient's dental insurance plan, and composites (plastic fillings), which have a one-third life expectancy of amalgam.

The conclusion that the ADA advances concerning dental mercury is that dentists and dental staff are within the safety zone of acceptability; that there is good evidence that mercury is not harmful because dentists and dental personnel have a higher exposure to mercury than do patients and there is no evidence that either group has a greater incidence of certain illnesses or a higher mortality rate than the general population. Furthermore, the ADA indicates that mercury levels found in patients are below that level found in dentists, and therefore, "patients are in no danger." The ADA concludes that ". . . [there is] no reason the average patient should seek to have amalgam restorations removed, unless hypersensitivity is evident."

## 3. QUICK REFERENCE OUTLINE (PRO-MERCURY)

(1) Sources of mercury exposure in the dental office
   a. Direct contact (handling) of mercury or mercury compounds during the fabrication of amalgam restorations.

    b. Inhalation of mercury vapors from
        1) contaminated office spaces as a result of
            a) accidental spills,
            b) leaking mercury dispensers,
            c) leaking or contaminated amalgamator capsules,
            d) the wringing of excess mercury after mixing the amalgam mass,
            e) vaporization of mercury from contaminated instruments placed in sterilizers,
            f) condensation of amalgam,
            g) improperly stored amalgam,
            h) organic mercurial disinfectants and
            i) contaminated amalgamators.
        2) the restorative process including
            a) the removal of the old amalgam restoration,
            b) the mixing of the new amalgam restoration,
            c) the placement of the new amalgam restoration and
            d) the carving and adjustment of the new amalgam restoration.

(2) Symptoms and injuries resulting from extremely high doses and/or chronic mercury exposure
    a. tremor (as seen in fine voluntary muscular movements, e.g. handwriting),
    b. loss of appetite,
    c. nausea,
    d. diarrhea,
    e. depression,
    f. fatigue,
    g. irritability,
    h. moodiness,
    i. pneumonitis,
    j. nephritis,
    k. nervous excitability,
    l. insomnia,
    m. headache,
    n. swollen glands and tongue,
    o. ulceration of oral mucosa,
    p. dark pigmentation of the marginal gingiva, and
    q. loosening of teeth.

(3) Symptoms or signs resulting from allergic reactions
    a. localized dermatitis
    b. generalized erythema.

(4) Biological responses: Bauer's paper[5] was quoted and was not qualified by the ADA
  a. Mercury is accumulated in the kidney, liver, brain and heart muscle.
  b. The central nervous system (CNS) is sensitive to mercury which is "related to high lipid content in, and slow elimination from, nervous tissue."
  c. The effect of mercury is to "block the metabolism of the neurons producing necrosis and irreversible damage."

(5) Mercury testing service available for dental staff
  a. Measurement of urine mercury levels
  b. Between January, 1982 and November, 1983, 776 dentists and staff were tested
    1) The average urine mercury level (dentists and staff) was 14.6 ug/l
    2) The average urine mercury for the general population is 3.0 ug/l
    3) Neurological symptoms are detected at 500 ug/l (another publication indicates 150 ug/l

(6) Health of dental staff (Shapiro's paper[12] was quoted and was not qualified by ADA)
  a. In an X-ray fluorescent study
  b. Of the 298 dentists, 23 had tissue mercury levels above 20 ug/g
  c. 30 percent of 23 had polyneuropathies
    1) some had electrophysiological abnormalities consistent with carpal tunnel syndrome (CTS)
    2) some had high visuographic dysfunction
    3) more "symptom-distress" than control group (those with less than 20 ug/g)

(7) Recommendations for the replacement of amalgam restorations
  a. A sound healthy tooth will suffer structural loss in removal of a restoration which can lead to the need for endodontic (root canal) therapy or the loss of tooth.
  b. Gold replacement wouldn't likely be covered by the patient's dental insurance plan.
  c. The composite life expectancy is about 5 years compared to amalgam which is about 15 years.

(8) Conclusion (ADA position)
  a. Dentists and staff are within safety zone of acceptability.
  b. There is good evidence that mercury is not harmful because dentists and dental personnel have a higher exposure to mer-

cury than patients and there is no evidence that either group has a greater incidence of certain illnesses or a higher mortality rate than the general population.

    c. The mercury levels found in patients are below that level found in dentists and therefore, "patients are in no danger."[3]

    d. ". . . no reason the average patient should seek to have amalgam restorations removed, unless hypersensitivity is evident."[4]

## 4. EVALUATION[2–4,6–11]

After evaluating the American Dental Association, pro-mercury position, I find that the ADA position has four major parts. First, the ADA acknowledges that dentists, dental personnel and patients are exposed to mercury vapor during the restorative process. They conclude that because dental personnel have used mercury for 150 years without ill effects, mercury is safe. This is a forceful argument if it is true. If mercury is toxic, the ADA argues that dental personnel would be the first to demonstrate symptoms of poisoning since their exposure to mercury is greater than the exposure of any dental patient.

Comprehensive studies were conducted at Temple University which measured the incidence of major diseases and mortality among dentists compared to the general population. The study measured the incidence of cancer, leukemia, diabetes, mental disorders, cardiovascular-renal diseases, non-malignant respiratory disease, cirrhosis, nephritis, and suicide. There was a statistically significant difference between dentists and the general population concerning cancer of the brain, cardiovascular-renal diseases, non-malignant respiratory disease, suicide, ill-defined causes of death and all other causes of death.[13] Although I cannot draw a causal connection between mercury exposure and these causes of death in dentists, three questions come to mind. Can the significant incidences of diseases of the brain, cardiovascular system, kidney and respiratory system be related to dentists' long-term occupational exposure to mercury since mercury either accumulates or passes through those tissues? Remember, the ADA's own study indicates an almost five-fold increase in urine mercury among dentists compared with the general population. Second, since acute or chronic exposure to mercury results in neurological symptoms, such as depression and tremor, can the long-term occupational exposure to mercury contribute to the high suicide rate among dentists? Third, can the statistically significant death rates from "ill defined causes" and from "all other causes" be related to the fact that chronic mercury exposure usually cannot be causally connected to specific signs, symptoms and diseases?

The second part of the ADA's position acknowledges that mercury can, in rare cases, result in hypersensitivity or allergy; a condition that "usually turns up as skin rash and is similar to other common allergies." The ADA states that the percentage of the population affected by these reactions is one percent. The ADA's acknowledgment that allergy or hypersensitivity to mercury exists is consistent with published scientific findings. However, the statement that mercury allergy is rare and is similar to other common allergies or hypersensitivities is misleading for two reasons. First, reading the listings in the *Index of Dental Literature* leads one to believe that allergy to dental amalgam is more common than one percent. Second, the ADA's use of such a narrow definition of allergy may lead the patient to believe that mercury allergy is limited to sneezing, itching or skin rashes. The symptoms and signs of mercury allergy as manifested in *only* local dermatitis and generalized edema[4] represents the traditional allergist's view rather than the broader definition of allergy embraced by the American Academy of Environmental Medicine. Modern scientific thinking has recognized a broader concept of allergy. Dr. Randolph describes the progression of an allergic reaction from mainly physical symptoms which are commonly recognized as an allergic reaction (runny nose, itching, hives) to systemic symptoms (fatigue, depression, headache).[14] These systemic symptoms had not been recognized as allergy prior to this expanded concept. The belief that an allergic reaction is an indication that the body is unable to adapt to something in its environment suggests that the maladaption may be manifested elsewhere in the body. If manifested somewhere else in the body, the maladaptive reaction could be considerably different from the expected common allergic response.

In addition to the allergic response, an inflammatory reaction may occur. Inflammatory reactions are general reactions which affect the entire body. The inflammatory response can produce localized edema (swelling) and toxicity. This toxic inflammation can compromise the healthy functioning of tissues because it causes tissue injury and increases the need for nutrients. Because of this tissue injury there is a good opportunity for infectious agents to injure the body or for additional maladaptive reactions to occur.[15]

The third part of the ADA's position is their view concerning the replacement of amalgam fillings. The ADA warns patients that structural tooth loss occurs during the replacement of amalgam. They also warn of the possibility of tooth devitalization during the restorative process and of the low life-expectancy of composite replacements. Each of these warnings is valid, but all of these warnings must be put into their proper perspective. Structural tooth loss occurs during tooth preparation for any type of filling. The more often your dentist has to replace your fillings, the more tooth structure he or she must remove in order to properly prepare the tooth for the new filling. A tooth may be devitalized (the nerve may die) not only during preparation for a filling but also because of extensive decay or trauma (injury). Finally, the life expectancy of composites refers to their having less strength than amalgams. While this may have been true in the past, the latest composite filling materials are approaching the strength of amalgam. In addition to composites and amalgam, gold is an excellent alternative.

Finally, the ADA cites the OSHA standard as a guideline for safe levels of mercury vapor within the dental office. The ADA uses the OSHA standard to demonstrate that because the concentration of mercury in the air of dental office is below the TLV, that dental personnel are not being exposed to unsafe amounts of mercury.[16] The OSHA standard (TLV = 50 ug/m$^3$) was established to protect industrial workers from "harmful" exposure to mercury in the work place. The basis for this figure was the standard set by the American Conference for Government and Industrial Hygienists and the American National Standard Institute (see Appendix II). When translated to the dental office, the TLV is misleading because the mercury levels in the dental office often exceed 50 ug/m$^3$ during the removal of a single amalgam restoration. A review of the literature indicates a difference of opinion about what level of mercury is considered safe: the Russian standard is a TLV of 10 ug/m$^3$ based on Trakhtenberg's studies;[17] the United States NIOSH standard is a TLV of 20 ug/m$^3$. This range from ten to fifty micrograms indicates that the experts are unsure about the safety of air mercury. Additionally, air mercury safety does not address the potential adverse effects of mercury compounds on dental personnel or patients because it does not take into account the health status or the individual susceptibility of the practitioner or patient.

A major weakness in the ADA's position is that it has not taken a more aggressive role in assessing the current scientific literature which suggests that dental mercury is harmful. Since the ADA is a representative body and is *the* authority on dental materials, its laissez-faire attitude will prevent dentists from trying alternative filling materials. Because of this laid-back attitude on the part of the ADA, the authority which it has enjoyed will likely be eroded. If this occurs, dentists and patients alike will suffer since there will no longer be a dependable and credible central dental authority. Finally, the ADA's attitude towards mercury can result in a casual attitude of practicing dentists which may harm the health of these dentists as well as their staff.

The ADA's argument to dissuade a patient from replacing fillings on the basis of non-insurance coverage shows an insensitivity to the health-conscious dental consumer and is a weak argument indeed. When a patient's health and wellbeing is at stake, insurance coverage is not generally a top priority.

## LOOKING BACK

*A SUMMARY OF THE ADA'S POSITION:*

1. Mercury has been used for over 150 years and is considered by the ADA to be safe.
2. The sources of mercury exposure are from direct contact, inhalation of mercury vapor and mercury compounds.
   a. This amount of mercury exposure is, except for office contamination, below the TLV and does not, therefore, result in mercury poisoning.
   b. At risk to this mercury exposure are dental personnel, not patients.
   c. The amount of mercury vapor found in dental offices has never been shown to be associated with various diseases or medical conditions.
   d. Physiological effects do not occur until urinary mercury levels reach 150 ug/l.
   e. Studies indicate that dental amalgam contributes little or no mercury to the body.
3. Dental personnel are a generally healthy group without ill effects from their contact with mercury.
4. Except for mercury poisoning, symptoms (reactions) to mercury result from allergic reaction manifested in localized dermatitis and generalized erythema. The ADA further estimates that less than 1 percent of the population is affected by mercury allergy.
5. Replacement of amalgam fillings is not advised unless there is documented evidence of sensitivity to mercury.
6. Effects of replacing amalgam fillings include structural loss of the tooth, devitalization and short life expectancy of composite replacement restorations. These factors should be considered prior to instituting treatment.

# REFERENCES

1. "Facts About States for the Dentist Seeking a Location," American Dental Association, Chicago, p. 8, 1982.
2. "Media Message Misleads," *ADA News* (Chicago), November 21, 1983.
3. "Dentists, Staff Members Healthy, Despite Daily Contact with Mercury," *ADA News* (Chicago), December 1983.
4. "ADA President Underscores Safety of Dental Fillings," *ADA News Bulletin*, 130a/83/JHB.
5. Bauer, J. and First, H.: "The Toxicity of Mercury in Dental Amalgam," *CDA Journal*, 10:47–61, June 1982.
6. "Mercury in the Office," *ADA News* (Chicago), November 21, 1983.
7. "Mercury Hygiene Measures Recommended," *ADA News* (Chicago), September 7, 1981.
8. "Recommendations in Dental Mercury Hygiene, 1984," Council on Dental Materials, Instruments, and Equipment, *JADA*, Vol. 109, October 1984.
9. "Safety of Dental Amalgam," Council on Dental Materials, Instruments and Equipment and Council of Dental Therapeutics, *JADA*, vol. 106, April 1983.
10. Rupp, N, and Paffenbarger, J.: "Significance to Health of Mercury Used in Dental Practice: A Review," JADA, 82(6):1401–1407, June 1971.
11. "Safeguarding the Physical Well-Being of Dentists," *JADA*, 110:15–24, January 1985.
12. Shapiro, I.: "Neurological and Neuropsychological Function in Mercury-Exposed Dentists," *Lancet*, May 22, 1982.
13. Orner, G. and Mumma, R.: "Mortality Study of Dentists," Temple University, Philadelphia, December 30, 1976.
14. Randolph, T. and Moss, R.: *An Alternative Approach to Allergies*, Lippincott and Crowell, New York, pp. 29–39, 1979.
15. Philpott, W and Kalita, D.: *Brain Allergies: The Psychonutrient Connection*, Keats Publishing, New Canaan, Conn., p. 103, 1980.
16. "Experts to Review Safety of Metals in Dentistry," *ADA News* (Chicago), December 1983.
17. Trakhtenberg, I.: *Chronic Effects of Mercury on Organisms*, (Translation by Fogarty International Center for Advanced Study in the Health Sciences), U.S. Dept. of HEW Public Service, National Institute of Health, D HEW Pub (NIH) 74-473, 1974.

# 7
# THE ANTI-MERCURY POSITION

LOOKING AHEAD

1. ANTI-MERCURY POSITION: BACKGROUND

2. THE ANTI-MERCURY POSITION

3. ANTI-MERCURY—QUICK REFERENCE OUTLINE

4. ANTI-MERCURY POSITION: EVALUATION

5. GENERAL ASSESSMENT OF THE ANTI-MERCURY POSITION

LOOKING BACK

## LOOKING AHEAD

The anti-mercury group believes that the mercury in dental fillings causes or contributes to a variety of diseases. The main spokesmen for this position are Sam Ziff and Dr. Hal Huggins. Sam Ziff publishes the newsletter, *Bioprobe, Inc.*, Orlando, Florida and is the author of *The Toxic Time Bomb*, a book which advocates the anti-mercury position. *The Toxic Time Bomb* discusses the use of mercury in dentistry, the forms of mercury and the biological mechanisms of mercury.[1] Mr. Ziff makes arguments against the use of mercury in dentistry using articles published by the ADA and other scientists. He discusses electricity in the mouth, the signs, symptoms and pathology of mercury poisoning and case histories. The book is basically a literature review containing case histories provided by dentists practicing mercury-free dentistry. Mr. Ziff's book contains clear and concise references to the scientific literature.

Dr. Huggins holds a D.D.S. degree from the University of Nebraska and is the author of *It's All in Your Head*, a book which promotes the anti-mercury position.[2] The companies with which he is affiliated are: Toxic Element Research Foundation (TERF), Matrix Minerals Inc. and Step Ahead Marketing, Inc. Dr. Huggins is located in Colorado Springs, Co. *It's All In Your Head* discusses the exposure to, biotransformation of and adverse effects of dental mercury, the diagnosis of and treatment for mercury toxicity, nutrition and supplementation. In addition, the book presents case histories from Dr. Huggins' dental practice. Dr. Huggins' comments are obviously one-sided. Two major flaws in his book are the use of incomplete references and the difficulty in determining what information is credited to which reference.

Toxic Testing, Inc., Altamonte Springs, Florida, a company which sells mercury toxicity products, is not affiliated with either spokesman.

This chapter discusses the arguments advanced by the anti-mercury spokesmen. *However, you should be aware that the individual dentists who practice mercury-free dentistry may differ in their approach, philosophy and adherence from the prescribed protocol of Mr. Ziff and Dr. Huggins.* Although this chapter evaluates the anti-mercury position in general, you are responsible for evaluating your dentist's approach.

## 1. BACKGROUND

The anti-mercury group (spokesmen for amalgam replacement) maintains that the mercury in amalgam fillings is poisonous to patients. They claim that mercury adversely affects the neurological system, the cardiovascular system, the connective tissue system and the immune system. It is their belief that mercury affects this wide range of biological systems because it blocks the action of *manganese* which is the chief mineral activator of these systems.

## 2. THE ANTI-MERCURY POSITION[1-3]

I have organized the anti-mercury position into twelve major categories. The topics I will discuss include:

(1) Conditions Necessary for Mercury to Cause a Problem
(2) Sources of Mercury
(3) Reactions to Mercury
(4) Fate of Mercury
(5) The Biotransformation of Mercury
(6) The Diagnosis of Mercury Toxicity
(7) Treating Mercury Toxicity
(8) Prognosis for Mercury Replacement
(9) Factors Which Determine Patient Improvement
(10) Patient Improvement After Amalgam Removal
(11) Supplementation Program
(12) Computer Analysis

(1) *Conditions Necessary for Mercury to Cause a Problem*—The anti-mercury group indicates that in order for the mercury in dental fillings to cause a problem for patients, four things must occur. First, mercury would have to come out of the filling. Second, this mercury has to be in high enough doses. Third, this liberated mercury would then have to form a compound that would be toxic. Fourth, the exposure to mercury would have to cause symptoms or conditions that go into remission upon removal of mercury.

(2) *Sources of Mercury*—Mercury is released as a by-product of electrical activity occurring in the dental amalgam filling. Dr. Huggins describes this electrical activity in two ways:

"One is like a standard battery. The two different metals in an electrolyte (solution that can conduct electricity) will produce a current (flow of electrons). This is called a bi-metallic cell. (The term "cell" refers to a minute area that produces electrical activity.) The other cell which exists on a filling . . . [is called] a differential aeration cell. . . . This refers to electrical activity that exists between two areas of saliva containing different amounts of oxygen."[4]

(3) *Reactions to Mercury*—Mercury from dental fillings can cause neurological reactions such as irritability, depression, suicidal tendencies, muscle spasms, seizures, facial twitches, and multiple sclerosis. It also can cause cardiovascular symptoms which include chest pains and rapid heart beat. The anti-mercury group also claims that mercury contributes to collagen diseases such as scleroderma, arthritis, lupus and bursitis and diseases of the immune system.

(4) *Fate of Mercury*—Mercury vapor enters the body by being inhaled into the lungs, by being absorbed by the lining of the nose and by being absorbed into the pulp of the tooth. Mr. Ziff indicates that from this entry into the body, mercury "travels by way of biological pathways" throughout the body by attaching to compounds normally found in the body. Mercury may remain in the body from a few days to twenty-two years.[5]

(5) *The Biotransformation of Mercury*—Mercury vapor which is liberated from dental amalgam fillings is methylated by *Streptococcus mutans* (a bacteria which lives on the surface of the tooth). This methyl mercury is 100 to 1,000 times as toxic as metallic mercury.

(6) *The Diagnosis of Mercury Toxicity*—The diagnosis of mercury toxicity involves the patient's answers to a questionnaire, an oral examination by the dentist, electrical testing with an amalgameter, mercury patch testing and blood, urine and hair analyses. AUTHOR'S NOTE: There are two types of patch tests: the "allergic eczematous contact dermatitis" patch test and the "provocative" patch test. The difference between the two is in what patient reactions are measured. The "allergic eczematous contact dermatitis" patch test is an objective test which measures the skin response of a patient to a given substance. The "provocative" patch test is a subjective test which measures both the skin response and the systemic response a patient has to a given substance. The anti-mercury group uses both approaches.

A different questionnaire is used by both Toxic Testing Inc. and by Dr. Huggins. Dr. Huggins' questionnaire is on page 51 of his book. Both questionnaires fundamentally seek the same information. This information ranges from whether the patient experiences simple indigestion to whether the patient has been diagnosed as having degenerative diseases such as diabetes and cancer.

The amalgameter is an instrument which measures the electric current generated within the metallic fillings in the mouth. The readings can range from positive to negative; negative readings are said to be more harmful. The higher the current [more negative], the greater the mercury loss. Dr. Huggins states that "the higher the electrical current, the faster the chemical reactions are taking place."[6] The amalgameter readings dictate the sequence by which amalgam fillings are removed; the most negative fillings are removed first.

Patients are also tested for mercury sensitivity using the mercury patch test. This test indicates whether a patient is allergic to mercury. An additional reason for a mercury patch test is to elicit those symptoms which are thought to be caused by dental amalgam.

Blood tests include a white blood count, red blood count and a serum analysis. The white blood count is said to be influenced by toxic metals. A high white blood count is suggestive of an acute reaction; a low white blood count suggests a chronic immune challenge. The red blood count as well as the hematocrit (the percentage of cells in a volume of blood) is raised by mercury. In addition, total plasma protein, globulin and albumin are measured to indicate the body's ability to process mercury-related antigens. The ratio of total protein/globulin is said to indicate the toxic status of the patient.

The patient's urine is tested for vitamin C levels which indicate the body's relative ability to dispose of mercury after the mercury has been released from storage. The urine is also tested for mercury levels, which demonstrate both mercury exposure and the body's ability to excrete mercury.

Hair analysis evaluates both the minerals and the toxic metals present in the hair.

(7) *Treating Mercury Toxicity*—Once it has been demonstrated through the questionnaire (presence of symptoms), by patch testing (allergy to mercury), by amalgameter testing (negative reading fillings), by urine screening (low or high mercury levels), that the patient is "mercury toxic" or allergic to mercury, the dentist recommends the replacement of amalgam fillings. The treatment plan includes recommended supplementation to help excrete the mercury contained in the tissues and the sequence to follow in removing the amalgams.

(8) *Prognosis for Mercury Replacement*—An 80 percent success rate is expected if the amalgam fillings are removed in the sequence indicated by the amalgameter readings *and* if the patient takes the prescribed supplements (supplementation is called "biochemical coverage").

(9) *Factors Which Determine Patient Improvement*—The factors which determine patient improvements are the same factors that are

indicated in the prognosis for mercury replacement: sequential amalgam removal and prescribed supplements.

(10) *Patient Improvement After Amalgam Removal*—The patient's symptoms that are said to improve after amalgam removal are: neurological reactions such as irritability, depression, suicidal tendencies, muscle spasms, seizures, facial twitches, and multiple sclerosis. In addition, cardiovascular symptoms which include chest pains and rapid heart beat are said to decrease. The anti-mercury group also claims that mercury removal positively affects the course of collagen diseases such as scleroderma, arthritis, lupus and bursitis and diseases of the immune system.

(11) *Supplementation Program*—The supplementation program proposed by the anti-mercury group has as its purpose the alteration of cell membrane permeability which helps mercury to be excreted from the body.

(12) *Computer Analysis*—Computer analysis offered by Dr. Huggins analyzes the results of blood, urine and hair testing and the nutritional status of the patient.

## 3. QUICK-REFERENCE OUTLINE

(1) Conditions Necessary for Mercury to Cause a Problem[7]
   a. Mercury must come out of the filling,
   b. The concentration of mercury should be high enough to produce ill effects,
   c. Mercury would form a compound that would be toxic
   d. Mercury exposure would form conditions that go into remission upon removal [of the amalgam fillings].

(2) Sources of mercury[8,9]
   a. Mercury is released from the tooth as a result of a "battery effect" as demonstrated in the reduction of the mercury content of five-year-old amalgams (28 percent vs 50 percent when new).

(3) Reactions to Mercury[10,11]
   a. Neurological
      1) emotional: irritability, depression, suicidal tendencies.
      2) motor: muscle spasms, seizures, facial twitches and multiple sclerosis.

b. Cardiovascular: alterations of heart performance (chest pains/ rapid heart beat).
c. Collagen diseases: scleroderma, arthritis, lupus and bursitis.
d. Immunological: defense system—antibodies and white blood cells.
e. Allergies: mercury in combination with what you are "allergic to" ruptures white blood cells and cause allergic reactions.

(4) Fate of Mercury[2,3,12]
    a. Mercury vapor is inhaled into the lungs and then travels into the blood stream.
    b. Mercury vapor goes into the brain via the nasal sinus through axonal transport.
    c. Mercury vapor elevates hemoglobin and hematocrit; oxygen transport is reduced causing fatigue.
    d. A fetus has higher mercury levels than the mother due to high amount of red blood cells (RBCs).

(5) The Biotransformation of Mercury[13,14]
    a. Mercury vapor from fillings is methylated by *Streptococcus mutans* (a bacteria which lives on the surface of the tooth).
    b. Methyl mercury is 100 to 1,000 times as toxic as elemental mercury.

(6) The Diagnosis of Mercury Toxicity[15]
    a. Diagnosis program
        1) questionnaire
        2) dentist does
            a) oral examination
            b) electrical testing with amalgameter
        3) blood analysis
        4) urine analysis
        5) hair analysis
    b. Diagnostic factors
        1) Complete blood count[16]
            a) white blood count (WBC) is sensitive to toxic metals (high = acute reaction; low = chronic immune challenge).
            b) red blood count: reduced by mercury.
            c) hemoglobin: reduced by mercury.
            d) hematocrit: reduced by mercury.
            e) efficiency of oxygen-carrying capacity is reduced by mercury.
        2) Blood profile[17]
            a) total protein, globulin and albumin indicate ability to process mercury-related antigens.

b) total protein/globulin ratio projects toxic status of the patient.
3) Hair analysis[18]
   a) evaluation of calcium, manganese and mercury.
4) Urine vitamin C[19]
   a) Shows relative ability of body to dispose of mercury after it has been released from storage.
5) Urine mercury
   a) Low levels indicate inability to excrete mercury resulting in mercury retention.
   b) High levels indicate:
      (a) high exposure or
      (2) body is dumping mercury.
6) Body temperature: not diagnostic at this time.
7) Electric current[20]
   a) The higher the current, the greater the mercury loss.
   b) Copper amalgams give off greater mercury than the current reading predicts.
   c) Negatively charged fillings are more damaging.
   d) Amalgameter—device to measure electrical current potential of fillings in teeth.[21]
      (1) Purpose—predict hypersensitivity and make treatment plan for mercury toxic patient.
      (2) Readings—10 microamps to 50 microamps
      (3) Use:
         (a) ground is placed under tongue
         (b) probe is placed on the filling
         (c) if no reading—polish or scratch surface to remove oxide layer.
      (4) Analysis
         (a) Multiple sclerosis patients have at least 6 negative fillings.
         (b) Cardiac patients have high positive fillings.
         (c) Negative reading is worst but prognosis is best.
         (d) Dycal (a calcium hydroxide liner put between the filling and the tooth) can cause symptoms similar to mercury toxicity in some patients.
         (e) The electric current created in dental materials can affect EKG and EEG.
      (5) Fluctations in readings due to:
         (a) freshness of the battery used in the meter
         (b) type of battery used in the meter

(7) Treating Mercury Toxicity
  a. Testing method
    1) Tests are conducted on patient's blood for immune reactions, red blood cell count and white blood cell count.
    2) Hair analysis for toxic metals and minerals.
    3) Urinalysis to determine amount of excreted mercury.
      a) If urine mercury is low—patient has difficulty excreting mercury and therefore, mercury is retained in the body. These are toxic patients.
      b) Mercury levels above 12 ug/l = patient is being exposed to above average amount of mercury but is able to excrete it.
  b. Testing for mercury sensitivity:
    1) Mercury sensitivity patch test.[22]
      a) Purpose: screening patients for probability of hypersensitivity to heavy metals. Not diagnostic of heavy metal toxicity by itself.
      b) Parameters:
        (1) blood pressure
        (2) pulse rate
        (3) onset of symptoms
      c) Contraindications
        (1) Patient with multiple sclerosis, seizures, or severe headaches.
        (2) Patient who is pregnant.
      d) Reading the patch test
        (1) Positive reactions produced by hypersensitive patients are 65 percent systemic and 35 percent local.
        (2) Positive reactions show:
          (a) changes in blood pressure
          (b) changes in pulse rate
          (c) changes in temperature
        (3) Most frequent positive signs and symptoms:
          (a) change in blood pressure
          (b) change in temperature
          (c) change in pulse
          (d) redness
          (e) itching or burning in area of patch
          (f) headaches
          (g) flu-like symptoms (weakness/tiredness)
          (h) cold hands and feet
          (i) light-headedness
          (j) nausea

(4) Patient is considered to have a positive reaction if during the first hour of the testing procedure:
  (a) Increase or decrease of 10 or more points in systolic
or diastolic blood pressure.
  (b) Increase or decrease of 10 or more points in pulse
rate.
  (c) Increase or decrease of 0.5 degrees in oral temperature.
 e) Contraindications for patch testing:
  (1) pregnancy
  (2) suicidal tendencies
  (3) seizures
  (4) multiple sclerosis
 f) Antidote for the patch test reaction: 6 grams of sodium
ascorbate powder in water.
2) Diagnosis of heavy metal toxicity made by interpretation of
body's reaction to heavy metal contamination revealed by:
 a) analysis of hair for heavy metals
 b) analysis of urine for mercury levels
 c) analysis of blood profile
 d) analysis of white blood count

(8) Prognosis for Mercury Replacement:
There is an 80 percent success rate if patient follows:
 a. Amalgam removal: must be done sequentially.
  1) first, remove high reading, negatively charged fillings.
  2) second, remove low reading, negatively charged fillings.
  3) third, remove high reading, positively charged fillings.
  4) fourth, remove low reading, positively charged fillings.
 b. Biochemical coverage.

(9) Factors Which Determine Patient Improvement[23]
 a. Sequential amalgam removal.
 b. Biochemical coverage.

(10) Patient Improvement After Amalgam Removal[24]
 a. Neurological.
  1) emotional—irritability, depression, suicide.
  2) motor—epilepsy, seizures, multiple sclerosis.
 b. Cardiovascular.
  1) tachycardia (rapid heartbeat).
  2) angina (unidentified chest pain).
 c. Collagen—arthritis, tennis elbow, scleroderma, lupus and
myofibrocytis.
 d. Allergy—food sensitivities, airborne allergies, universal reactors.

e. Immune system—white blood cells, alteration of differential, reduced hemoglobin oxygen-carrying capacity.

(11) Supplementation Program[25]
a. Purpose:
   1) To change cell membrane permeability (facilitates passage of oxygen into cell and carbon dioxide out of the cell).
   2) To chemically process mercury after it is out of the cell (facilitate excretion of mercury from the body).
b. Dr. Huggins' supplementation schedule—begins several days prior to amalgam removal.

(12) Computer Analysis[3,26]
a. Urinary screening program: measures mercury levels in urine.
b. Mercury Toxicity Diagnosis Program: analysis of blood, urine and hair mercury levels.
c. Nutritional Evaluation Report: nutritional evaluation and planning.
d. Mercury Toxicity Comparison: follow-up program.
e. Special Analysis: analysis by Doctor Huggins.
f. BCI, Jr: an introduction to mineral analysis.
g. BCI Professional Blood Analysis: a guide to nutrition.
h. BCI Professional Hair Analysis: a guide to counseling patient on minerals.

## 4. EVALUATION[1,2,3]

During my evaluation of the anti-mercury position, I refer to the scientific literature, which is presented and documented in Chapter Eight, The Literature Review. After evaluating the information presented by Mr. Ziff and Dr. Huggins, I find that the anti-mercury position can be divided into four major parts:

1. The Hypothesis (Topics #1,2,4,5 Listed in the Anti-Mercury Position)
2. Patient Reactions to Mercury Toxicity (Topic #3)
3. Diagnosis of Mercury Toxicity (Topic #6)
4. Treatment and Prognosis (Topics #7,8,9,10,11,12)

1) The Hypothesis: The anti-mercury position maintains that in order for the mercury in dental fillings to cause a problem for patients, four conditions must occur: mercury must leave the amalgam filling, the mercury liberated by the amalgam filling must be in high enough doses, the mercury would have to form a compound

that would be toxic, and the mercury would have to cause symptoms that go into remission upon its removal.

The first condition, that mercury must leave the amalgam filling, is supported by scientific literature. Studies have shown that mercury is liberated from an amalgam filling during chewing, through corrosion and through absorption into the pulp of the tooth.

The second condition, that the liberated mercury must be in a high enough dose, is vague. The spokesmen do not make a clear distinction between acute and chronic exposure and they do not openly recognize the significance of biological differences among individuals. As you saw in Chapter Two, Toxicity, there are two types of toxicity: acute and chronic. An acute exposure is a high dose of toxin at one time; a chronic exposure refers to smaller amounts over a long period of time. I assume that the spokesmen for the anti-mercury position are referring to chronic toxicity. I agree that in order to have a toxic reaction, a person would have to be exposed to mercury in a high dose for that individual; whether it is an acute or chronic exposure. In chronic exposure, the individual's reaction is important because the dose of mercury can be very small and yet be toxic. The difficulty in evaluating exactly what dose is high enough is that toxicity has many facets:

1. The Nature of the Toxin—How toxic is the substance?
2. The Dose of the Toxin—How much toxin are you exposed to?
3. The Duration of the Toxin—Is the exposure acute or chronic?
4. The individual's susceptibility—How does your body deal with the toxin?
5. The Route of Entry—Can the toxin get to where it can do harm?
6. The Additive Effects of the Toxin—What is the total body burden of toxins?

At this point, I will further clarify the inherent character (nature) of toxins. Mercury vapor is toxic, but is less toxic than methyl mercury. The reason for this is in the characteristics of the mercury molecule itself. Methyl mercury is 100 to 1,000 times more toxic than mercury vapor. This means that we can expect at least 100 molecules of mercury vapor to be about as toxic as one molecule of methyl mercury. Both Mr. Ziff and Dr. Huggins talk about the effects of mercury exposure as if both mercury vapor and methyl mercury were one and the same. I can understand why they group them together; their basic premise is that the mercury vapor liberated from dental amalgam fillings is converted to methyl mercury. I do not agree with this "grouping" approach because they have not established that methylation of mercury occurs in the body and, if methylation does occur, that the methyl mercury is present long enough to cause damage. Let's separate the literature according to experiments involving mercury vapor (mercury ions) and methyl mercury. Remember, a large part of experimentation is done on single celled organisms or animals. In the published literature, it is

METHYL MERCURY that impairs the incorporation of amino acids into brain tissues.
METHYL MERCURY that causes more extensive structural damage to the brain.
METHYL MERCURY that changes metabolic responses of the brain.
METHYL MERCURY that causes neurological damage.
METHYL MERCURY that interferes with vision.
METHYL MERCURY that interferes with message transmission by nerves.
METHYL MERCURY that affects electrocardiographs.
METHYL MERCURY that causes stress intolerance, low fertility and decreased sexual activity in animals.
METHYL MERCURY that causes damage to the chromosomes of the white blood cells.

As far as proving that mercury vapor is biotransformed to methyl mercury, both Mr. Ziff and Dr. Huggins cite a study by Heintze[27] to support their case. In this study, it was determined that certain bacteria found in the mouth (*Streptococcus mitior*, *Streptococcus mutans* and *Streptococcus sanguis*) could methylate mercury in the laboratory. Heintze indicated that "the results [of our experiment] indicate that organic mercury compounds may be formed in the oral cavity [mouth]." Heintze continued later in the article to say that ". . . several strains of bacteria and yeasts are capable of degrading methyl mercury to inorganic mercury." In an article cited by Heintze, Hidemitsu[28] indicates that a single strain of bacteria is able to convert mercury vapor to methyl mercury and, on the other hand, is also able to convert methyl mercury to mercury vapor.[27] The fat that both reactions can occur within the same strain of bacteria certainly weakens the case presented by Mr. Ziff and Dr. Huggins.

The third condition, mercury forms a compound that would be toxic, is misleading. Mercury vapor itself is toxic without having to form any additional toxic compounds. The anti-mercury group also indicates that the mercury vapor released from dental fillings is converted (biotransformed) into the *more* toxic methyl mercury. This is the cornerstone of the anti-mercury argument: that the primary problem with amalgams is the conversion of mercury vapor to methyl mercury. It is true that mercury is toxic and that some forms of mercury are more toxic than others. If the mercury vapor is in fact converted (biotransformed) to methyl mercury, then their case is stronger. If mercury vapor is not converted or if another mechanism demethylates (converts methyl mercury back to mercury vapor) methyl mercury before any damage is done, their case is weakened. The literature supports the opinion that mercury vapor is converted to methyl mercury; however, the literature also supports the fact that methyl mercury is demethylated back into metallic mercury. Both reactions occur in laboratory experiments. There is no scientific proof that either reaction occurs in humans.[29]

Finally, the anti-mercury position maintains that symptoms caused by mercury toxicity would have to be reversed upon removal of the amalgam fillings. If there were no permanent damage to the body and the symptoms expressed by the patient were due *only* to mercury exposure from his or her dental fillings, this opinion may be true. However, if toxicity from mercury exposure caused permanent injury to cells or tissues, there would only be a limited reversal of symptoms. In addition, this statement leads the reader to believe that mercury from dental fillings is the *only* cause for the indicated symptoms and then assumes that these symptoms will go away if the amalgam fillings are removed. An exact relationship between *only* mercury exposure from dental amalgams and a particular symptom has not been scientifically established. The decrease in symptoms may be attributed to patient improvement resulting from the recommended diet (no refined carbohydrate, alcohol, chocolate, margarine, soft drinks or cigarettes), the recommended vitamins or from decreasing the total body burden of toxins as a result of removing the amalgams. I am not comfortable with this single cause-effect reasoning, because current medical thinking is recognizing that many factors, working together, contribute to disease. The anti-mercury thinking eliminates other important factors which may contribute to the patients' symptoms and runs the risk that the patients will look no further in their attempt to achieve optimum health.

Both Mr. Ziff and Dr. Huggins indicate that the mercury from dental amalgams enters the body through the lungs and through the dental pulp. This is supported by scientific literature.

2) Patient Reactions to Mercury Toxicity: The anti-mercury position maintains that the mercury from dental fillings causes or contributes to a wide range of diseases. They assert that the common denominator among these diseases is that mercury blocks the action of manga-

nese in the body. I have been unable to find any scientific proof that connects mercury with manganese in causing diseases.

However, recent research has indicated the importance of minerals in relation to the toxic products produced by bacteria. Researchers have found that a common and usually harmless bacterium called *Staphylococcus aureus* produced up to twenty times as much toxin as usual when magnesium was removed from the bacterium's environment.[30] You can readily see that if mercury does interfere with certain minerals, it may indirectly cause disease. If you cannot supply the friendly bacteria in your system with the proper nutrients that they need, they will not function properly and may inadvertently add to your toxic load. What we are seeing in this case is that bacteria that do not receive proper nutrients produce excess toxins. Can we speculate that if humans do not get proper nutrients, they may produce a greater amount of toxins and thereby stress their biological systems?

The available literature does indicate that mercury has a chemical attraction for sulfur, nitrogen, oxygen and the halogens (chlorine, bromine, iodine); this chemical combination may interfere with body processes.

Other heavy metals are also known to cause health problems. *Time* magazine ("Putting the Knock on Lead") related a directive by the Environmental Protection Agency (EPA) to oil refiners.[31] The EPA told refiners that they must eliminate 90 percent of lead added to gasoline. The EPA stated:

> ". . . lead poisoning can damage the brain, liver and kidneys, particularly in children. Recent studies have linked lead to high blood pressure. . . . the EPA estimates that the cut back [of added lead] could prevent some 5,000 heart attacks and 1,000 strokes next year alone."

Because lead and mercury are both heavy metals and produce similar reactions, we may find that mercury also is involved in cardiovascular disease.

3) Diagnosis of Mercury Toxicity: The diagnosis of mercury toxicity advocated by the anti-mercury group includes a questionnaire, an examination by the dentist, electrical testing with an amalgameter, mercury patch testing and blood, urine and hair analyses.

Mr. Ziff and Dr. Huggins claim that the mercury liberated from dental amalgam is biotransformed into methyl mercury and interferes with body processes. In order to demonstrate this toxicity, Dr. Huggins recommends blood studies which generally evaluate the patient's blood chemistry as well as the patient's blood level of mercury. He relates the results of blood chemistry analyses to mercury toxicity. Dr. Huggins also recommends testing other components of the blood which are not diagnostic for mercury toxicity at the present time.

Urine mercury analysis is recommended by Mr. Ziff and Dr. Huggins as a preliminary screening test; they also use it later in treatment as a test to determine the individual's ability to excrete mercury. Dr. Huggins concludes that urine mercury levels indicate one of two things: low urine mercury levels demonstrate that the individual is unable to excrete mercury, whereas high urine mercury levels indicate either a high exposure to mercury or that the body is "dumping" mercury. I see a third possibility. Low urine mercury levels may indicate either no exposure to mercury or such a low exposure that the mercury level cannot be measured.

Hair analysis is used to determine hair mercury levels as well as the levels of minerals. The use of hair analysis to measure heavy metals is broadly accepted by the scientific community; on the other hand, using hair analysis to indicate the level of minerals in the body is controversial, but gaining acceptance.

4) Treatment and Prognosis: I will discuss both treatment and prognosis in the same section since they are related. The anti-mercury spokesmen indicate that in 80 percent of the cases, successful elimination of symptoms depends on: 1) sequential removal of amalgam fillings and 2) the use of prescribed supplements to allow the body to excrete mercury. I am assuming that adherence to the prescribed diet is also essential.

Once it has been established that the patient is allergic to mercury (via patch test) or that the mercury in dental amalgams is toxic (via amalgameter readings, blood, urine and hair analyses), a decision is made to replace the amalgam fillings.

The protocol for treatment of mercury toxicity is as follows:

1. Establish the sequence for amalgam removal using the amalgameter
2. Prescribe supplements
3. Remove the amalgam fillings according to the sequence indicated by the amalgameter readings.

Because of Dr. Huggins' theory that negative fillings cause symptoms, it is his recommendation that amalgam fillings be removed according to the following sequence:

1) First, remove high-reading negatively charged fillings.
2) Second, remove low-reading negatively charged fillings.
3) Third, remove high-reading positively charged fillings.
4) Fourth, remove low-reading positively charged fillings.

The recommended protocol for amalgam removal is first to re-move the quadrant of amalgams containing the filling with the most negative reading without regard to the readings of adjacent fillings. (AUTHOR'S NOTE: Your teeth are horizontally divided into upper teeth and lower teeth. Each of these sections is further vertically divided in half into right or left sides. Each of the four sections is called a quadrant. Therefore, you have an upper right quadrant, an upper left quadrant, a lower right quadrant and a lower left quadrant.)

*Figure 2:* **How teeth are divided into quadrants**

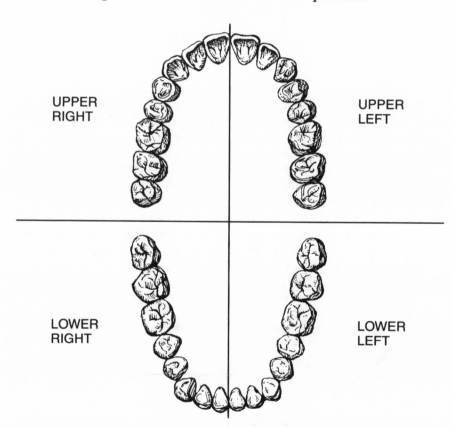

UPPER RIGHT      UPPER LEFT

LOWER RIGHT      LOWER LEFT

The relationship of the electric current reading and the order of amalgam removal is not supported by the literature.[32,33] If the electric current theory is correct, the amalgam removal should take place in the exact order indicated by the amalgameter readings of the fillings; that is, the most negative filling first, followed by the second most negative filling, regardless of where those fillings are located with respect to quadrants. To remove *all* amalgams in a quadrant at the same time, on the basis of finding the one amalgam with the most negative reading in that quadrant, appears to be inconsistent. Additionally, Dr. Alsoph Corwin (Professor Emeritus of Chemistry) of Johns Hopkins University has stated:

> "[I have been] unable to find any documented data to support such a protocol [sequential removal of amalgam fillings]. It has not been established whether the toxic agent in mercury poisoning from amalgam fillings is mercury vapor or dimethylmercury. In either case, the removal of the source of intoxication should benefit the patient, regardless of the sequence of removal of the fillings."[34]

Supplementation with vitamins and minerals is begun before dental treatment is started. The purpose of this supplementation program is threefold: to encourage the excretion of mercury from the cells, to prevent exacerbation of symptoms and to provide the patient with a nutrient base for rebuilding damaged body tissues.

In addition to vitamins, minerals and mercury-related supplements, Dr. Huggins recommends hormone supplements, lithium and protamine zinc insulin.

Health professionals generally agree that supplements should be prescribed for patients who demonstrate a need for such supplements. There is less agreement, however, in what levels of nutrients are needed and what steps will be taken to meet those needs. The range of opinions varies from the most conservative approach (individual approach) to the least conservative ("shotgun") approach. The conservative protocol would be to assess the patient's need for vitamins, minerals, amino acids and fatty acids through blood and urine tests. Once the patient's needs are determined, *only* those nutrients which are needed are prescribed. For example, if it were demonstrated by blood tests that there was a deficiency of vitamin B1, only B1 would be prescribed, not a B-complex vitamin. As you can see, this is a highly individualized approach to supplement therapy.

The shotgun approach to supplementation is to prescribe high doses (megadoses) of vitamins and minerals on the belief that food does not provide all the nutrients that we need and that we will excrete most excess vitamins. This is the least individualized approach to supplements, and some scientists believe that it may do more harm than good since fat soluble vitamins tend to accumulate in your body.

Dr. Huggins' supplementation program appears to fall in between the two extremes and is probably suitable for many patients. However, I disagree with Dr. Huggins' supplementation program for two reasons: he assumes that all patients are able to tolerate the supplements necessary for cell membrane conditioning and for mercury excretion and his use of some "supplements" clearly belongs in the realm of medicine.

First, Dr. Huggins assumes that all patients are able to tolerate the prescribed supplements. Although the description of his vitamins lists the contents, it does not indicate the food source from which each vitamin was derived. The average patient may not have a problem with this, but, according to physician and patient answers submitted in response to my surveys (Chapter Nine), one of the biggest problems that patients had during amalgam removal was with the prescribed supplements. Of course, the patients I refer to are not average patients. They have acute allergies and/or chemical sensitivities. I believe that there are many patients who can benefit from knowing the food sources of the vitamins they take and who would be better able to select individually tolerable brands of vitamins. I wrote to Dr. Huggins requesting information on food sources for his vitamins and was not able to obtain that information. His letter stated that the vitamins ". . . are as allergy-free as can be." For these reasons, I must recommend caution for allergic or chemically sensitive patients in their choice of vitamins and formulations.

My second area of disagreement with Dr. Huggins is with his use of "supplements" which clearly belong in the medical field. Dr. Huggins uses hormones, protamine zinc insulin (long-acting diabetes medicine) and lithium (anti-depressive medication) in treating the mercury-toxic patients. The use of these preparations leads me to question whether the improvement seen in some patients is from the amalgam removal or from the "supplements." For example, if the treatment plan for a depressed patient includes both lithium medication and amalgam replacement, how can you determine which treatment relieved the depression?

Toxic Testing Inc. recommends supplements which contain a combination of vitamins, minerals and amino acids. Toxic Testing Inc. has two supplement kits: one is their standard kit and the other is a "yeast-free" kit. Both are said to contain "special vitamins/

minerals, enzymes, amino acids, herbs, glandulars and co-factors to detoxify mercury/nickel and other heavy metals." Toxic Testing Inc. also does not identify the food source of its vitamins. In addition, they use "dl" methionine which contains the biologically inactive "d" methionine. These vitamins may be less expensive, but are more wasteful, since some of the product is not used by your body.

Both Mr. Ziff and Dr. Huggins recommend vitamin C for the treatment of mercury toxicity. They recommend vitamin C (sodium ascorbate) to "neutralize" a reaction caused by the exposure to mercury and to help excrete mercury from the body. The use of vitamin C in mercury toxicity is supported by independent scientific research. (Dr. Philpott related a study in which guinea pigs, given the human equivalent of 14 g of ascorbic acid daily, were protected from death from what should have been a fatal dose of mercury.[35])

Neither of the anti-mercury spokesmen recommend the use of essential fatty acids in their supplementation program. Essential fatty acids (EFAs) are important in the formation of prostaglandins. Prostaglandins are hormone-like substances which your body produces. The prostaglandins are important in a wide variety of metabolic processes. Some of these processes include: participation in anti-inflammatory reactions, regulating blood vessels, relaxing bronchial smooth muscle, regulating the immune system and regulating the use of insulin. Your physician can order laboratory tests to determine if you have a deficiency of essential fatty acids.

## 5. OVERVIEW

On the positive side, the anti-mercury spokesmen have made a contribution to health by identifying and making the public aware of the exposure to and potential effects of mercury; namely, the mercury vaporization from dental amalgams and the way mercury can potentially interfere with bodily processes. The anti-mercury group has put to good advantage the published accounts of mercury toxicity, mercury allergy and the potential effects of mercury on the body's biochemical systems, and have incorporated various testing procedures to support their hypothesis that mercury is liberated from dental fillings and can therefore be toxic to the patient.

On the negative side, the anti-mercury spokesmen give the impression that they believe the symptoms which they have identified are caused *only* by mercury exposure and that only amalgam replacement will alleviate these symptoms. Both Mr. Ziff and Dr. Huggins draw a parallel between the introduction of amalgam to dentistry and the appearance of new diseases spanning a period of nearly 100 years. This correlation between the introduction of amalgam to dentistry and the identification of specific diseases during that time period is circumstantial and not conclusive, as there are many factors other than mercury to consider.[36]

Dr. Huggins claims an 80 percent success rate in eliminating patient symptoms. This success depends on the patient following each of his recommended procedures: having amalgams removed in the order dictated by the measurement of electric current using the amalgameter, and taking supplements from his affiliated vitamin company.[37]

In conclusion, the anti-mercury spokesmen should be credited for their persistence in attempting to inform organized dentistry, the dental profession and the public of the dangers of mercury in dental amalgam. Because their hypotheses of the biotransformation of mercury to methyl mercury in humans and the need for the sequential removal of amalgam fillings have not been scientifically proven does not diminish the value of their warnings about dental mercury. My greatest reservation about their position is that it focuses too greatly on mercury as *the* toxin. A more acceptable approach is to focus on the effect of toxins in general and place mercury in its perspective.

## LOOKING BACK

### SUMMARY OF THE ANTI-MERCURY POSITION

1. Mercury is a poison.
2. Mercury accumulates in the body.
3. Mercury is biotransformed in the body into methyl mercury by certain bacteria.
4. Dental mercury causes or contributes to many diseases because mercury blocks the action of manganese which is the common link among many bodily processes.
4. Diagnosis for mercury toxicity includes a questionnaire; electrical readings (amalgameter); blood, urine and hair analysis; skin patch testing.
6. Treatment includes:
   a. Supplementation.
   b. Sequential amalgam removal according to current readings.
   c. Diet control.
7. Improvements are said to include symptoms in the neurological, cardiovascular, collagen and immune systems.

# REFERENCES

1. Ziff, S.: *The Toxic Time Bomb*, Aurora Press, New York, 1984.
2. Huggins, H. and Huggins, S.: *It's All in Your Head*, Colorado Springs, Colorado, 1985.
3. Huggins, H.: "What is Mercury Toxicity?," Basic Information Packet, Colorado Springs, Colorado, 1984.
4. Huggins, H. and Huggins, S.: *It's All in Your Head*, Colorado Springs, Colorado, p. 27, 1985.
5. Ziff, S.: *The Toxic Time Bomb*, Aurora Press, New York, 1984, pp. 71–82.
6. Huggins, H. and Huggins, S.: *It's All in Your Head*, Colorado Springs, Colorado, 1985. p. 67.
7. *Ibid.*, p. 19.
8. *Ibid.*, pp. 23–32.
9. Ziff, S.: *The Toxic Time Bomb*, Aurora Press, New York, pp. 65–70, 1984.
10. Huggins, H. and Huggins, S.: *It's All in Your Head*, Colorado Springs, Colorado, pp. 37–45, 1985.
11. Ziff, S.: *The Toxic Time Bomb*, Aurora Press, New York, pp. 83–110; 119–125, 1984.
12. *Ibid.*, pp. 71–82.
13. Huggins, H. and Huggins, S.: *It's All in Your Head*, Colorado Springs, Colorado, pp. 29–31, 1985.
14. Ziff, S.: *The Toxic Time Bomb*, Aurora Press, New York, pp. 30–33, 1984.
15. Huggins, H. and Huggins, S.: *It's All in Your Head*, Colorado Springs, Colorado, pp. 49–72, 1985.
16. *Ibid.*, pp. 60–61.
17. *Ibid.*, p. 56.
18. *Ibid.*, p. 60.
19. *Ibid.*, pp. 78–82.
20. *Ibid.*, pp. 25–27.
21. *Ibid.*, p. 52.
22. *Ibid.*, p. 53.
23. *Ibid.*, pp. 110–112.
24. *Ibid.*, pp. 37–47.
25. *Ibid.*, pp. 79–97.
26. *Ibid.*, p. 73.
27. Heintze, U., Edwardson, S., Derand, T. and Birkhed, D.: "Methylation of Mercury from Dental Amalgam and Mercuric Chloride by Oral Streptococci in Vitro," *Scand J Dent Res*, 91(2):150–152, April 1983.
28. Hidemitsu, S., Pan-Hou, H., Honsono, M. and Imura, N.: "Plasmid-Controlled Mercury Biotransformation by Clostridium cochlearium T-2," *Applied Environ Micro*, 40(6):1007–1011, December 1980.
29. Gabuten, G., Personal Communication, FDA, Rockville, Md., March 22, 1985.

30. "The Magnesium Connection," *Time*, p. 77, June 17, 1985.
31. "Putting the Knock on Lead," *Time*, p. 46, March 18, 1985.
32. Huggins, H. and Huggins, S: *It's All in Your Head*, Colorado Springs, Colorado, pp. 67–72, 1985.
33. *Ibid*.
34. Corwin, A., (Professor of Chemistry, Emeritus, Johns-Hopkins University), Personal Communication, June 1, 1985.
35. Philpott, W. and Kalita, D.: *Brain Allergies: The Psychonutrient Connection*, Keats Publishing, Inc., New Canaan, Connecticut, pp. 90–93, 1980.
36. Huggins, H. and Huggins, S.: *It's All in Your Head*, Colorado Springs, Colorado, p. 45, 1985.
37. *Ibid.*, p. 37.

# 8
# THE LITERATURE REVIEW

LOOKING AHEAD

1. BACKGROUND

2. LITERATURE REVIEW: EXPOSURE TO MERCURY

3. LITERATURE REVIEW: TOXICITY

4. LITERATURE REVIEW: ALLERGY

5. SYSTEMIC DISEASES RELATED TO MERCURY

6. AMALGAM REPLACEMENT IN THE LITERATURE

7. EVALUATION OF SCIENTIFIC LITERATURE

LOOKING BACK

# LOOKING AHEAD

Two graduate students, one from the Department of Audiology (sound) and one from the Physics department, decided to conduct an experiment about the reaction of frogs to various stimuli. They took elaborate steps to design the experiment which was to measure the distance a frog could jump with missing appendages (legs). They marked off the distance in which the frogs could jump in centimeters. They decided to allow three jumps per set of experiments and the average of the three jumps would be the result for that set. They then went out to find frogs with missing legs. After a lot of searching, they finally found a representative for each of the five categories they included in their experiment.

This is how the experiment went. The frog was placed at the start line, then one of the students would, at the same time, yell "JUMP!" and slap his hand on the table. When the frog jumped, the distance was measured and recorded. This experiment was first conducted with the frog having all four legs. The frog was placed on the starting line, the student yelled "JUMP!" and slapped his hand on the table. The distance jumped by the four-legged frog was measured and recorded. This procedure was repeated until all frogs had three chances to jump. The results were as follows:

1. When jump is yelled, and the table is slapped, the frog with all four legs jumps 150 cm.
2. When jump is yelled, and the table is slapped, the frog missing the left front leg jumps 125 cm.
3. When jump is yelled, and the table is slapped, the frog missing the left and right front legs jumps 120 cm.
4. When jump is yelled, and the table is slapped, the frog missing both front legs and the left rear leg jumps 50 cm.
5. When jump is yelled, and the table is slapped, the frog missing all legs did not jump at all.

After much deliberation the two students were having a difficult time making a conclusion. The audiology student concluded that since the frog with no legs did not jump when he yelled "JUMP!" frogs without legs cannot hear. On the other hand, the physics student concluded that the frog without legs did not jump because it could not feel the vibration of the slap on the table. In desperation, they turned to a fellow student who was a psychology major for advice.

After the three students repeated the experiment, the psychology student observed that the frog without legs looked and acted depressed and obviously had deep psychological problems. He concluded that the frog did not jump because he was probably rebelling against the experimenters.

While this story is facetious, it does illustrate a couple of points. The first point is that we usually judge things in our environment according to our experiences. Conclusions are drawn according to the individual's training. If you are a virologist (scientist who studies viruses), you might look into the possibility that viruses cause cancer; if you are an immunologist, you might look into the possibility that a faulty immune system causes cancer.

The second point is that sometimes a physician may give up on a patient as a result of his frustrated attempts to find a physical basis for his patient's complaints. Often, under these circumstances, the physician will refer the patient to a psychiatrist or psychologist more out of desperation than as a part of diagnosis and treatment. A psychological evaluation when used in conjunction with a physical examination is greatly effective in many situations because there is often a psychological component to disease.

While you are evaluating the review of the literature it is important that you realize that the experimenters are human. They solve problems according to their training and their perspective.

## 1. BACKGROUND

Each time you go to the dental office, you are exposed to mercury. This mercury exposure comes from mercury vapor in the office air, mercury vapor produced by the removal of old amalgam fillings, and mercury vapor produced by the insertion of new amalgam fillings.[1-4] This chapter contains an outline of articles appearing in the literature which describe the exposure to mercury, the toxic and allergic potential of mercury and its compounds. The literature review contains numerous studies about mercury toxicity and mercury allergy (hypersensitivity). You should be aware that these two areas sometimes overlap.

There are two types of information available about mercury exposure. The first type comes from studies conducted on individuals who have been exposed to mercury through accident or occupation. Examples of this are the Minamata Bay disaster and the Iraqi disaster discussed in Chapter Four. This information is extremely reliable since the observations were made on humans. Included in this type of information are human case histories and human group experiments which were known not to be harmful. The second type of information about mercury comes from experiments conducted in the laboratory. Many of the scientific experiments discussed in this chapter were done in vitro; that is, experimentation done on single-celled organisms and on animals in the laboratory in an artificial environment. While laboratory experimentation reveals the potential for certain reactions, it cannot be assumed that all reactions which occur in vitro (in the laboratory) also occur in vivo (in the human body). Therefore, the second thing which you must keep in mind is that some of the in-vitro experiments only indicate the *potential* for adverse effects on humans. Since we cannot experiment with toxins in humans, this in vitro experimentation is our best second choice. This chapter presents the information published in dental, medical, science and occupational journals and books on the exposure to mercury and its potential adverse effects.

## 2. LITERATURE REVIEW: EXPOSURE TO MERCURY

When we discuss exposure to mercury, we speak in terms of measurements. As you saw in Chapter Four, the terms gram, liter and meter are used to describe these measurements. In order to simplify your understanding of the measurements used in each study and to help you to compare studies, I have converted all measurements to micrograms (ug).

Weight conversion values:
  1 gram (g) = 1,000 milligrams (mg)
  1 milligram (mg) = 1,000 micrograms (ug)
  1 microgram (ug) = 1,000 nanograms (ng)

### A. Standards for Air Mercury

The Threshold Limit Value (TLV) is used to measure the "safe" levels of mercury in the workplace. This measurement is the maximum exposure to mercury vapor which is not harmful over a series of five daily exposure periods of eight hours each during a one-week interval. The TLV varies according to the values accepted by researchers, government agencies and by different governments themselves. Since there is no agreement among researchers, agencies and governments, the TLV may not be a reliable standard. For example, the TLV for mercury in the United States is five times that accepted in the USSR.

Accepted TLV Standards (see Appendix II):
  Air mercury vapor levels:

  (1) TLV = 50 ug/m$^3$ (OSHA)[5]
  (2) TLV = 20 ug/m$^3$ (NIOSH)[5]

(3) TLV = 10 ug/m$^3$ (USSR)[5]
(4) PEL = 50 ug/m$^3$ (California ISHA)[6]
(5) "Ceiling limit" = 100 ug/m$^3$ (short term exposure)[6]
(6) TWA (time weighted average) = 6 ug Hg/100 ml of blood corresponds to a time weighted average air exposure of 100 ug Hg/m$^3$[7]

## B. Instruments Used to Measure Mercury Vapor

There are two instruments used to measure mercury vapor; the Backarack and the Jerome.[7] The Jerome instrument is considered to be a more reliable indicator of mercury in the air. Doctors Cooley and Young have cautioned against the use of these instruments to indicate the need to replace amalgams.[7] They state that "due to the variables and uncertainties involved, oral measurements obtained with [these] instruments should not be related directly to the patient's health."

1) Backarack Mercury Sniffer
   Manufacturer: Backarack Instrument Co., Pittsburgh, Pa.
   Description: Chamber with ultraviolet light on one end and photoelectric cell on the other end.
   Shortcomings: Also sensitive to organic acids, dust, cigarette smoke and water vapor.
   Recommendations: Not accurate for use in the mouth.

2) Jerome Mercury Vapor Analyzer
   Manufacturer: Jerome Instruments, Jerome, Arizona
   Description: Absorption of mercury on thin gold film.
   Shortcomings: Cost ($4000)
   Recommendations: Measurement of mouth mercury with this device should not be related to health of the patient.

## C. Exposure to Mercury Vapor

As you have seen before, you are exposed to mercury each time you visit the dental office. In addition to this exposure, you are exposed to mercury vapor during the removal of an amalgam filling and during the placement, wear and corrosion of that amalgam filling.

1) *Office air mercury levels*: The air in the dental office contains mercury vapor because approximately 75 percent of the fillings that

the average dentist uses are amalgams. Because of this extensive use and the high volatility of mercury, it is practically impossible to avoid some air contamination. Dentists are concerned about the concentration of mercury vapor in their offices. OSHA and NIOSH have established Threshold Limit Values. The TLV was established to protect employees from the harmful effects of toxins.[5] As we discussed before, the TLV varies among agencies and among countries. The United States' TLV is the highest concentration of air mercury considered "safe" among the major world powers.

2) *Mercury exposure during amalgam removal:* During the removal of amalgams, the patient is exposed to mercury. This exposure has been documented through urine mercury levels before removal, immediately after removal (urine mercury = 6 ug/l) and for several days after removal.[8] The studies indicated that soon after the removal of amalgam fillings, the urine mercury level increased but tapered off to pre-removal levels within a few days.

3) *Mercury exposure during amalgam placement:* The literature indicates that the patient is exposed to mercury vapor during the placement of amalgam fillings.[9,10] Air mercury levels can reach as high as 100 ug/m$^3$ during the process of mixing and placing amalgam fillings.[8,10] Setting amalgam was determined in the laboratory to emit a detectable amount of mercury vapor into the air for 400 minutes. Researchers estimated this level to be 1.2 ug/square centimeter of amalgam surface at 37°C (when the temperature of the amalgam was raised to body temperature).[11]

4) *Subsequent mercury exposures:* In the past, amalgam was thought to be inert; that is, no mercury was liberated by dental amalgam. The reasoning behind this was that the mercury in dental amalgams was quickly bound to the other metals. This binding was considered to be so stable that not even an amount of free mercury sufficient to cause allergic reactions could be given off.[10] More recently, this has been demonstrated not to be true. Researchers have found that mercury is liberated during chewing,[6,11–15] that mercury exists in the soft tissues adjacent to amalgam fillings[16,17] and that mercury is present in the dental pulp within 10 days after the placement of an amalgam filling.[10,18]

Gingival tissues adjacent to class V fillings (those along the gum line) have been shown to contain high amounts of mercury (147 ug/m$^3$ vs 3.0 ug/m$^3$ in an area not adjacent to amalgam).[16,17] The amount of mercury vapor depends on the type of alloy used and the amount of mercury in the placed amalgam filling.[13] The amount of mercury exposure is continuous throughout the patient's lifetime (prenatal and after).[12] In another study, it was determined that when the subjects swallowed amalgam particles that those amalgam particles liberated mercury. These swallowed amalgam particles resulted in urine mercury levels of 20 ug/l.[8]

5) *Corrosion of the amalgam filling:* Over time, all amalgam fillings corrode. This corrosion results in the liberation of mercury vapor.[19,73] This liberation of mercury vapor is accelerated if the patient has gold fillings, gold crowns or gold prosthetic devices (gold partial dentures and gold bridgework). Chewing also increases the amount of mercury vapor given off by the filling.[12,15,20–24] Studies have demonstrated that the corrosion of amalgam occurs from both the surface and the interior of the amalgam filling.[19]

Jaro Pleva, Ph.D., a corrosion chemist, researched dental amalgam and indicated that all amalgam corrodes. This corrosion liberates mercury vapor which is then inhaled through the lungs, ingested through the GI tract and absorbed through the teeth. Dr. Pleva's analysis of old (5 to 20 years old) amalgam fillings (using JEOL scanning electron microscope with EDAX—Energy Dispersive Analysis with X-rays) demonstrated a loss of mercury from these amalgam fillings in the range of 10 to 45 percent. He concluded that even "a very limited corrosion might be unacceptable when the released metal is highly toxic."[73]

6) *Mercury vaporization during chewing:* Chewing has been shown to cause volatilization of mercury from amalgam fillings.[6,11–15] This information is important because it illustrates that patients can be exposed to mercury vapor during chewing and during clenching or bruxing (grinding) their teeth. This volatilization has been demonstrated by the following experiments:

In the first experiment, forty-eight patients participated. Forty had amalgam fillings and eight had no amalgam fillings.[12] The following are details of the experiment:

a) Mouth mercury vapor was measured at rest (before chewing) and was found to be in the range of 0.10 to 2.16 ug/m$^3$.
b) Mouth mercury vapor was measured after chewing for 10 minutes and was found to be in the range of 0.08 to 87.5 ug/m$^3$.
c) The difference in mouth mercury vapor indicated that mercury was liberated during chewing. The average mouth mercury vapor increased 15.6-fold after chewing. This experiment

demonstrated that patients with amalgam fillings are exposed to mercury from their amalgam fillings during chewing.

Fifty patients participated in the second experiment in order to determine how much mercury exposure a patient received during chewing.[6] The following is a summary of the experiment:

a) Mouth mercury vapor was measured at rest and was found to be in the range of 0 to 3.0 ug/m$^3$.
b) Mouth mercury vapor was measured after chewing gum and was found to be in the range of 25 to 400 ug/m$^3$ (most common was 50 to 150 ug/m$^3$).
c) Vaporization of mercury is 45 ug/day (based on 10 teeth each with 0.1 ug/m$^3$ and chewing for 60 minutes/day).
d) The researcher indicated that the patient would have to excrete 45 ug/day to balance intake of mercury resulting from chewing.

The third experiment involved twenty pedodontic (children) patients who did not have fillings, but needed fillings.[12] The details of the experiment are as follows:

a) Mouth mercury vapor was measured at rest and was found to equal 0 ug/m$^3$.
b) Ten patients were given amalgam fillings; ten were given composite (plastic) fillings.
c) The amalgam group had a significant increase in mouth mercury vapor immediately after placing the fillings and a significantly higher mouth mercury vapor (during a chewing experiment) one week later than they did before the amalgam fillings were placed.

7) Conclusions on the effect that chewing has on mercury exposure:

a) The amount of liberated mercury vapor is related to size, number and mercury content of the completed amalgam fillings and the length of chewing time.[11–15]
b) Chewing removes the protective oxide formed on the surface of the amalgam filling.[25]
c) The amalgam fillings do not have to be in contact with each other to produce mercury vapor.
d) The increase in mercury vapor after chewing was an average of 15.6-fold over the prechewing mercury vapor levels.[12]

e) The amount of mercury liberated could be as much as 30 mg to 560 mg over a period of time depending on the size and the number of amalgam fillings,[22] but it has been suggested that this amount is about equal to the amount ingested in food (25 ug/day).[23,24] AUTHOR'S NOTE: The amount of mercury attributed to a person's diet would depend on what that individual eats.

f) Moisture was previously believed to prevent vaporization. This has been shown not to be true.[6] (Mercury amalgam submerged in water liberated from 600 to 1,000 ug/m$^3$ of mercury vapor.)

### D. Biotransformation of Mercury Vapor

Documentation of the biotransformation of mercury vapor is found in the scientific literature. Mercury vapor is biotransformed in vitro (in the laboratory) into methyl mercury by organisms normally found in the mouth. These organisms are *Streptococcus mitor*, *Streptococcus mutans* and *Streptococcus sanguis*. Since these organisms are found in bacterial placque, the white sticky substance that forms on your teeth, it has been suggested that this methylation process may also occur in the mouth.[26,27] Mercury vapor is also biotransformed into methyl mercury by human intestinal bacteria.[28]

On the other hand, a demethylation reaction, the biotransformation of methyl mercury to inorganic mercury, also occurs. As you saw in Chapter Seven, two reactions are possible: the methylation of mercury vapor to form methyl mercury and the demethylation of methyl mercury to form mercury vapor. Both of these reactions can be produced by the same strain (family) of bacteria.[29,30] In order to assess the accumulation of methyl mercury from mercury vapor, autopsies were performed on mercury miners. If mercury vapor was converted to methyl mercury in the body you would expect to find an accumulation of methyl mercury in these miners. This was not the case. There was no mercury accumulation found during autopsy.[31] There are two possible explanations for this data: either no mercury vapor was converted to methyl mercury or an equal amount of methyl mercury was converted back to mercury vapor so as to have a net amount of zero.

### E. Absorption of Mercury

1) *Mercury Vapor*—Mercury can be absorbed into the body through the lungs, skin, or GI tract. Mercury vapor is inhaled into the lungs.[8] Once in the lungs, mercury vapor is rapidly absorbed. Of

this amount, as much as 74 percent is retained by the lungs.[17] Seven percent of the 74 percent is released from the body through expired breath. This mercury vapor has a half-time of 18 hours. (Half-time means that at the end of a certain period of time, half of the amount of substance is lost. For example, if you were exposed to 100 atoms of mercury vapor, in 18 hours you would still have 50 atoms left in your body. Eighteen hours after that, you would have 25 atoms left, and so on).[17] Exhaled mercury vapor is considered to be an index of a recent exposure to mercury vapor.[17] Within 10 minutes, 30 percent of the inhaled mercury vapor is transferred to the blood.[8] Mercury vapor is poorly absorbed in the GI tract.[8,32]

2) *Mercury Salts*—Although mercury salts are absorbed in the GI tract, they are usually not of concern to the dental patient because the patient is exposed to mercury vapor both in the dental office and through the wear and corrosion of amalgam fillings.[32] However, mercury vapor is chemically converted to mercury ions in the blood. These mercury ions are the same ions as are found in mercury salts. Therefore, exposure to either mercury vapor or mercury salt results in the same product: mercury ions.[32] Some of the ingested mercury ions bind to the lining of the GI tract and to the contents of the intestine; some of the mercury ions enter the blood.[33]

3) *Organic mercury (methyl mercury)*—Methyl mercury is absorbed in the GI tract[32] and is 100 to 1,000 times more toxic than mercury vapor.[6]

### F. Measurements of Mercury Exposure

The exposure to mercury can be determined by three methods— blood mercury, urine mercury and hair mercury analyses. The "normal" limits of these three methods are outlined below:

a. Blood mercury levels[7]

Upper "normal" limit: 1.0 to 3.0 ug Hg/100ml of blood
   (95 percent contained less than 3.0 ug Hg/100ml of blood,
   1.2 percent contained 5-10 ug Hg/100ml of blood)

b. Urine mercury levels[7]

Upper "normal" limit (with occupational exposure): 0 to 30 ug Hg/l
Upper "normal" limit (without occupational exposure): 0 to 10 ug Hg/l

Urine mercury has little value in the diagnosis of mercury poisoning.[2,31]

Mercury is found in urine for up to 8 days after placing an amalgam filling.[34]

If urine mercury levels are:[7]
a) 100 ug Hg/24 hours—patient needs corrective action.
b) 200 ug Hg/24 hours—patient should be removed from the exposure.
c) 300 ug Hg/24 hours—patient has possible mercury poisoning.

c. Hair mercury levels ("normal")[7]

Men: 0.5 to 18.0 ug/g of hair
Women: 18.9 to 25 ug/g of hair

In a study comparing the amount of mercury in the hair to the amount of fish eaten, it was found that the amount of hair mercury increased with the amount of fish eaten.

The results are indicated below:

Fish consumed vs hair mercury levels[7]

a) When fish was eaten once/month: there were 1.4 parts of mercury per million parts of hair (ppm)
b) When fish was eaten once/2 weeks: hair mercury levels were 1.9 ppm
c) When fish was eaten once/week: hair mercury levels were 2.5 ppm
d) When fish were eaten once/day: hair mercury levels were 11.6 ppm

## G. The Chemistry of Mercury

Once mercury enters the blood, three reactions are possible: mercury may change oxidation state, mercury may combine (bind) with organic or inorganic ligands or mercury may accumulate in some cell organelles.[25] A change in oxidation state means that mercury would change from mercury vapor to mercuric ions. Combining with ligands means that mercury may attach to either organic compounds such as hemoglobin or inorganic compounds such as chlorine. The third possibility is the accumulation in one or more of the parts of the cell itself. Once in the blood, mercury vapor can be oxidized to mercuric ions within the blood or mercury vapor can be oxidized within the tissues. Of the amount of mercury oxidized in the blood, 16 percent is oxidized in the plasma—50 percent bound to hemoglobin and 50 percent bound to plasma albumin (protein)—and 84 percent is oxidized in red blood cells (there is 5 times the concentration of mercury in hemoglobin than in the plasma).[32,35]

### H. The Circulation of Mercury

The blood-brain barrier is a mechanism by which the blood vessels in the brain selectively keep certain materials from entering the brain cells. The placenta is the organ which allows the exchange of nutrients and waste materials between the fetus and the mother. The placenta has a membrane, the placental membrane, which acts in a similar way to the blood-brain barrier. Both mercury vapor and methyl mercury can cross the blood-brain barrier and the placenta.[32] Mercuric ions do not cross the blood-brain barrier or the placenta.[32] The literature indicates a significant correlation between stillbirths and mercury levels found in maternal and umbilical cord blood.[36] Because mercury vapor crosses both the blood-brain barrier and the placental membrane, it is wise to avoid entering the dental office unnecessarily during pregnancy since your exposure to mercury vapor may also expose your developing child to mercury.

### I. The Distribution of Mercury

Once in the body, mercury is distributed through most tissues; but, because of its affinity to certain chemical groups, mercury accumulates in the brain, kidney and liver. Some mercury vapor enters the brain before it is oxidized to mercuric ions. Mercuric ions are concentrated in the kidney.[32]

### J. The Excretion of Mercury

Mercury vapor is excreted by the lungs, in the urine and in the feces. Mercury ions are excreted in the urine and feces. Organic mercury (methyl mercury) is excreted in the feces.[32]

## 3. LITERATURE REVIEW: TOXICITY

### A. Adverse effects of mercury

1) *Background*: There is a wide variety of physical and chemical injuries that can lead to either acute or chronic inflammation and result in death of the cell. [33,37–39] Only a small number of mercuric

ions are necessary for cellular damage to occur. AUTHOR'S NOTE: a numerical value for the term "small" is not given by the researcher.[40] However, it is documented that mercury vapor of 1 to 10 ug/m$^3$ was sufficient to cause mercury poisoning in researchers.[41] Research has shown that ionic solutions (solutions containing the ion form of metals) in the concentration range of 10 to 4 to 10 to 6 of most metals composing dental amalgam inhibited amino acid incorporation into protein-like material of cells grown in laboratory culture.[40]

2) *Biochemical adverse effects:* Mercuric ions interact with sulfhydryl (-SH) and disulfide (-SS) groups in a multitude of biological systems to alter the function of these systems,[42] but the bonds formed by mercury and these groups are reversible.[2] Mercuric ions react with the sulfide (-S) groups in proteins[34] and with the sulfide groups of saliva amino acids.[34] Mercuric ions:

inhibit enzymes,[42,43]
inhibit urease, invertase and other enzymes containing sulfhydryl (-SH) groups,[34]
inhibit collagen synthesis by fibroblasts or epithelial cells,
may add to increased loss of the peridontal attachment (attachment of the gum to the tooth) seen adjacent to defective amalgam fillings,[19]
cause changes in cell membrane permeability,[6]
interact with enzymatic reactions in cells because of an affinity for nervous tissue,[34]
block metabolism of neurons producing irreversible nerve damage or necrosis (death)[44] and
block nerve conduction.[34]

Mercury bonds with ligands (compounds) and thus changes membrane permeability for nutrients and interferes with enzymes. *The damage to cells is dependent on the amount of mercury accumulated and the sensitivity of the individual.*[2]

3) *Toxic effect of mercury:* The toxic effect that mercury has on the body is related to rate and method of uptake by the blood.[35]

Whole blood uptake: 0.5 ug/hour/ml
Plasma uptake: 0.11 ug/hour/ml
Hemoglobin uptake: 1.0 ug/hour/ml

In order to determine if the level of mercury in expired air (mouth air mercury levels) and the level of blood mercury levels had any correlation, the following experiments were undertaken.[45]

## Table 2: SUMMARY OF THE FATE OF MERCURY:

| Forms | Ingestion | Distribution | Excretion | Crosses Brain or Placental Barriers | Test | Half-Time |
|---|---|---|---|---|---|---|
| Vapor | lungs | brain kidney | lungs urine feces | yes | urine | 65 days |
| Inorganic | GI tract | kidney | urine feces | no | urine | 65 days |
| Organic | GI tract | RBC's | feces | yes | RBC conc. | 65 days |

In the first experiment, 47 male medical students (with amalgams) and 4 medical and 10 graduate students (without amalgams) were examined. The results of this experiment are as follows:

|  | Mouth air mercury | | Mean blood-mercury levels |
|---|---|---|---|
|  | *Before chewing* | *After chewing* | |
| Amalgams | 0.00224 ug | 0.01897 ug | 0.0007 ug/ml |
| No Amalgams | 0.00113 ug | 0.00106 ug | 0.0003 ug/ml |

The conclusion drawn by the scientists was that the mercury that volatilized from the amalgams was inhaled and reached the blood via the lungs.

In a second experiment, a causal relationship between amalgam and blood mercury levels was found.[12] The details of the experiment were:

(a) After getting a base line blood mercury level, all amalgams were removed.

(b) Blood tests were performed at various intervals over the next 214 days.

(c) After day 57 there was a statistically significant reduction in blood mercury.

(d) Blood level at day 214 was 10 times below preremoval level.

The conclusion drawn by the researchers was that, for this patient, there was a causal relationship between dental amalgams and blood mercury levels.

## 4. LITERATURE REVIEW: ALLERGY

### A. Allergy to Mercury

1) *General mercury allergy:* The reactions that the body has in response to mercury can be either toxic or allergic. As you have seen, the immune system plays a role in disabling toxins; it also plays a role in providing your body with protection from foreign substances (antigens—which are usually proteins) by producing antibodies against that foreign substance. Therefore, a foreign substance can be both a toxin and, at the same time, stimulate your body to produce antibodies against it. Because both of these responses can

occur together, it is difficult to determine whether a specific response is a toxic response or an allergic response. For example, an inflammation of the skin can be caused by a toxin or by an allergic reaction.

On a cellular level, mercuric ions stimulate lymphocytes to revert back to immature forms.[46] Mercury allergy is latent (not showing) in healthy and non-allergic individuals.[47] Sensitivity is most frequent after amalgams have been in the mouth more than 5 years.[47] There is a considerable difference in the incidence of allergic reactions between healthy people and allergic patients.[47] The typical patient history of an allergy to mercury may include:[47–54]

a) Old amalgam fillings are replaced or new amalgam fillings are placed.
b) Within hours or days, the patient experiences edema (swelling) and urticaria (on the lips, tongue, face, neck, eyes, temples, upper back, chest or legs).
c) One case attributed allergic reaction over a 20-year period to the local anesthetics which were given before restorative procedures. The history revealed that the rashes occurred during amalgam placement and not during routine examinations. After twenty years, an amalgam was done without anesthetic. The rash occurred leaving the dentist to conclude that it was the amalgam and not the anesthetic agents causing the allergic response.[54]
(d) Some symptoms persist until the offending amalgam is removed.[53]

2) *Patient's history:* Items in a patient's history which may lead to suspicion of mercury sensitivity include (these may be with or without apparent symptoms):

a) Use of contraceptive jelly (phenylmercuric salt).[53]
b) A history of mercury on a ring resulted in "water blisters."[51]
c) Use of eye ointment (with mercuric oxide) without apparent reaction—may have sensitized patients without signs.[54]
d) Merbromin applied to a mosquito bite.[55]
e) Allergy to merthiolate or diuretics.

3) *Dental treatment for mercury-sensitive patients:* Antihistamines generally clear the allergic reaction if used systemically or locally.[51] If it is decided to use amalgam on mercury-sensitive patients, allergic reaction to mercury could be suppressed by antihistamines and careful technique.[51] Some eruptions do not resolve until all

amalgam contact is eliminated.[22,48] Because there is no significant difference in mercury patch test results between patients with amalgam fillings and those without fillings, mercury sensitivity appears not to be related to amalgams.[56] In laboratory experiments, the following metals were shown to cause immunosuppression:[57] mercury, copper, manganese, cobalt, cadmium, chromium, tin and zinc.

### B. Local allergic reactions

Allergy to mercury is one of the most common causes of dermatitis.[58] Dermatitis is an inflammation of the skin. Among the symptoms of mercury allergy are a rash appearing on the face the day following the placement of a dental amalgam filling,[51] fever and dermatitis several hours after the placement of a dental amalgam filling,[52] eczema, erythema and irritation several hours after the placement of a dental amalgam[54] and edema of the lips, chin and eyes 9–10 hours after amalgam placement followed by a rash of the neck, chest, thighs, popliteal fossae, forearms, antecubital fossae and hands.[53] Mercury hypersensitivity is specific for the epidermis because the antigen formed has protein conjugates present only in the epidermis.[53] Patients who had allergic contact dermatitis due to mercury can have skin lesions exacerbated by systemic administration of mercury.[53] After removal of amalgams, dermatitis was most pronounced on the side of the body on which mercury patch tests or amalgam fillings had been placed.[50]

### C. Oral manifestations of mercury allergy

1) *Signs and symptoms:* Signs and symptoms of mercury allergy can occur both on the skin and in the oral cavity.[59] The corrosion products of dental amalgam may retard the healing or modify repair of inflamed and healing gingival tissues (gums). This interference with healing and repair may complicate the management of gingival and periodontal disease.[60]

2) *Case Study:* A case history demonstrating the effect of amalgam fillings on peridontal health appeared in the literature. In this case, the patient had a history of high blood pressure, ulcers, hypo/hyperglycemia, anemia, vitamin deficiency (all vitamins), sulfa drug sensitivity, barbiturate sensitivity and aspirin sensitivity. In addition to these symptoms, the patient related a history of swollen ear lobes and finger rash caused by silver earrings. The patient's amalgam fillings were replaced and her peridontal condition resolved.[61]

## D. The effect of mercury on T lymphocytes[62]

1) Dental amalgam and nickel alloys can adversely affect the quantity of T lymphocytes. This finding is significant because abnormal T lymphocyte percentages or malfunction of T lymphocytes can increase the risk of cancer, infection and autoimmune diseases.

2) In the following study, tests were done to measure the T-cell percentage in relation to amalgam and nickel:

a) Patient #1 was asymptomatic 21-year-old female
   (1) Before treatment (had amalgams) T-cells: 47 percent
   (2) After removal of amalgams: T-cells: 73 percent
   (3) Change: +55.3 percent
   (4) After re-inserting amalgams: T-cells: 55 percent
   (5) Change: –24.7 percent
   (6) Remove the amalgams and insert gold fillings: T-cells: 72 percent
   (7) Change: +30.9 percent

b) Patient #2 was asymptomatic 20-year-old male
   (1) Before treatment (had composites): T-cells: 63 percent
   (2) After placing nickel alloy: T-cells: 56 percent
   (3) Change: –11 percent
   (4) Removal of nickel alloy: T-cells: 77 percent
   (5) Change: +37.5 percent

c) Patient #3 was 35-year-old female with multiple sclerosis
   (1) Before treatment (had amalgams): T-cells: 60 percent
   (2) After replacement of amalgams with gold: T-cells: 71 percent
   (3) Change: +18.3 percent
   AUTHOR'S NOTE: There was no mention of the patient's symptoms.

### E. Mercury patch tests

The use of a patch test to determine mercury sensitivity is indicated when mercury is suspected, but not known, to be the cause of an allergic reaction.[63]

1) Indications for use of a patch test:
   a) Cause of allergic contact dermatitis is unknown.
   b) Suspected responsible agent is unavoidable.

2) Contraindications:
   a) Presence of acute or widespread dermatitis.
   b) Suspected agent is corrosive or systemically toxic.
   c) During systemic corticosteroid treatment.
3) Site of application:
   a) Upper area of the back on either side of the vertebral column.
   b) Lateral aspects of upper arms.
4) Test agent concentration:
   a) If the concentration is too high:
      (1) False positive interpretation is possible.
      (2) Sensitization of the patient may occur.
   b) If the concentration is too low:
      False negative interpretation may occur.
5) Vehicles (the carrier of the agent) to avoid: substances which are irritants or common sensitizers (e.g. chloroform, benzene, turpentine, lanolin and some alcohols) should be avoided because of the confusion over whether the substance tested or the vehicle used caused the reaction.
6) Vehicles which are acceptable: aqueous for testing nickel and petrolatum for testing mercury (see discussion).
7) Read after 1 hour, 24 hours and 48 hours
8) Reevaluate after 4th or 5th day
9) Complications:
   a) Irritant reaction
   b) Vehicle is sensitizing
10) Situations for false positive reactions:
    a) Concentration of test material is too high
    b) Dermatitis is present
    c) Amount of test material is too large
    d) Reaction to vehicle or tape
    e) Wrong anatomical area for test
    f) Improper reading time
11) Situations for false negative reactions:
    a) Concentration of test material too low
    b) State of allergy is low
    c) Amount of test material is too low
    d) Wrong test material composition
    e) Improper vehicle
    f) Wrong anatomical area
    g) Improper reading time
12) Shortcomings to the patch test:
    a) Irritants resemble allergic reactions
    b) Vehicles may produce irritant reaction
    c) Subjectivity of clinician

13) Additional parameters (anti-mercury group):[64,65]
    a) Change in blood pressure
    b) Change in pulse
    c) Change in temperature
    d) Subjective signs such as cold or tingling hands or feet, headache, nausea, indigestion, sinusitis and depression
14) Miscellaneous:
    a) Prick test using mercury ammonium chloride and 1 percent mercuric oxide has been successful in testing sensitivity to mercury.[54]
    b) The American Dental Association recommends:[66]
        (1) Patients with suspected hypersensitivity should be referred to an allergist or dermatologist.
        (2) Procedure be performed by clinician professionally trained and experienced in administering and interpreting patch tests.

## 5. SYSTEMIC DISEASES RELATED TO MERCURY EXPOSURE

### A. Multiple Sclerosis (MS)[67]

1) Factors which may lead to development of MS:
    (a) Slow, retrograde seepage of ionic mercury from root canals or class V fillings inserted many years ago.
    (b) Recurrent caries (decay) and corrosion around filling edges
    (c) Oxidizing effect of the purulent (pus) response
2) Lead may act interchangeably with mercury
3) Unilateral MS derived from amalgam fillings in ipsolateral (same side) teeth
4) Generalized MS may result from
    (a) Ingestion or inhalation of volatile mercury
    (b) Inhalation of exhaust fumes of lead additives in gasoline

### B. Antibiotic resistance in bacteria

Mercuric ions induce antibiotic resistance in bacteria.[68]

### C. Lichen planus

Lichen planus is a shiny flat-topped eruption.

1) If positive patch test for mercury, removal of all amalgams are recommended in oral lichen planus.[69]

2) An increase in the incidence of allergic reactions to dental materials in lichen planus patients indicate that substances in dental materials may be of significance in cases of oral lichen planus.[70]

## 6. AMALGAM REPLACEMENT IN THE LITERATURE

A. Precautions to take when removing amalgams:[49]
   1) Use a rubber dam when removing amalgam fillings.
   2) Use adequate high speed suction when removing amalgams.
   3) Use phrophylactic antihistamines to minimize allergic reactions.
B. Primary decay should be treated with porcelain, silicate or gold.[50]
C. Amalgam fillings can be placed in mercury-allergic patient if amalgam is carefully handled and prophylactic administration of antihistamines is given.[51]
D. Removal of all amalgams should take place as soon as possible.[71]
E. Amalgam should be replaced with gold, porcelain or silicate when defects arise.[44]
F. Conventional composites are generally suitable for posterior fillings (molars).[49]
G. Microfine composites are better than conventional composites.[49]

## 7. EVALUATION OF THE SCIENTIFIC LITERATURE

Because of gaps in the literature, diverse opinions and some confusing published data, I have indicated some important notes to clarify the literature review.

1. Measurements, like statistics, are not conclusive on an individual basis. Adverse reactions could result in an individual patient from measurements of toxins well below what is considered the "safe" level.

2. As I discussed in the evaluation of the pro-mercury position, the safe levels of air mercury are speculative as indicated by the range of TLVs accepted by various researchers, government agencies and among different governments themselves. There is, however, a correlation between elevated mercury levels of blood and urine and elevated mercury levels in the air, but there is no correlation between these mercury levels and adverse symptoms. This seems to indicate that blood and urine mercury testing to

confirm a patient's symptoms is futile. A patient can have symptoms in spite of "normal" measurements for the levels of mercury in the blood and urine.

3. An individual's *recent* exposure to mercury can be indicated through studies of blood and urine. Measurements on a group basis are more reliable than those on an individual basis since the concentration of mercury in the blood or urine does not necessarily reflect the concentration of mercury in critical organs. The relationship between mercury intoxication, the concentration of mercury in tissues and the patient's symptoms are not dependent upon one another. On an individual basis, blood mercury levels are more reliable than urine mercury levels. Hair mercury, although not diagnostic, will give an indication of mercury exposure on a longer-term basis. Since the growth rate of hair is between 1 to 1.5 cm/month, some attempt can be made to obtain a history of mercury exposure.

4. Distribution of mercury in high amounts occurs in the kidney, liver, brain and heart muscle.[32] Excretion takes place through the lungs (mercury vapor), in the urine and in the feces. The half-time for the elimination of mercury is approximately 65 days with the exception of the brain which is 18–22 years.

5. In addition to the mercury exposure from air, food and water, exposure to mercury on a long-term chronic basis can occur through the wear and corrosion of amalgam fillings. This is demonstrated by the accumulation of mercury in soft tissues adjacent to amalgam fillings,[16] accumulation of mercury in the pulp of vital teeth,[10,18] the analysis of the mercury content of older fillings and the measurement of mercury vapor liberated from the filling after chewing.[11–15] The amount of mercury vapor released from fillings is inceased up to 15.6-fold by chewing.[12]

6. The fact that biotransformation of mercury vapor to methyl mercury takes place in the laboratory by certain human oral[26] and human intestinal[27,28] bacteria only *suggests* that methylation may be possible in the body. Although the extent of biotransformation is unknown, autopsies of mercury miners showed no methyl mercury accumulation.[31] Additionally, there is evidence that de-methylation also occurs by the same strain of bacteria.

7. The potential adverse effects of mercury toxicity include inflammation[37–39] and interference with certain biological systems. This interference is related to mercury's affinity for sulfur-containing

groups such as sulfhydryl (-SH) and disulfide (-SS).[34,42] There is also the potential for interference with the sulfur-containing amino acids cysteine and methionine. [8,40,72] Sulfhydryl groups are contained in glutathione, cysteine, coenzyme A, lipoamide, urease, invertase and mercaptans.[34] Mercaptan is the sulfur-containing compound which is used in pesticides and fungicides; it is also the substance added to natural gas to give it its characteristic odor. Disulfide groups are contained in cystine.

8. The affinity that mercury has for nervous tissue affects the enzymatic reactions in that tissue[34] and blocks the metabolism of neurons.[44]

9. Mercury may systemically affect an individual in multiple sclerosis[67] and lichen planus.[69,70] Mercury also induces resistance to antibiotics in bacteria.[68]

10. Reported mercury allergy is manifested *both* locally (dermatitis) and systemically (erythema).[51–54,58,59]

11. The typical history for a patient with mercury allergy would include a sensitizing experience of which the patient may or may not be aware.[47–55] Experiences such as the use of mercuric salts in the form of creams,[55] eye ointments,[54] contraceptive jellies[53] or contact lens solutions with a mercuric preservative are noteworthy. At some time later, an amalgam filling is placed and within hours to days the patient experiences one or more of the following signs: fever, urticaria of lip, tongue, face, neck, eyes, temples, upper back, chest or legs, dermatitis or rash on the face or legs.[71]

12. Patch testing for mercury sensitivity is indicated when allergy or hypersensitivity is suspected but not known.[63] The test is composed of objective and subjective parameters and is best done by someone trained and experienced in allergy testing. Care must be taken to assure that the vehicle used does not produce an allergic reaction on its own.

13. The use of antihistamines during placement or removal of amalgams or to eliminate allergic reactions has been suggested.[49,51] This suggestion will be effective if the patient's symptoms are due to a true allergy to mercury. I question the concomitant use of amalgam and antihistamines to suppress symptoms of mercury allergy. Relief from the cause of allergy appears to be the prudent choice.

14. A more important area covered in the literature is the potential effect of mercury on the immune system. As important as is the typical allergic reaction (rash, hives and itching), more important are mercury's potential short- and long-term effects on the function of the immune system. Mercury's interference with the immune system may lead to more serious and debilitating conditions. Dental amalgam and nickel alloys have been shown to affect the quantity of T lymphocytes. Abnormal T-cell percentages or malfunction of T-cells can increase the risk of cancer, infection and auto-immune diseases.[62]

## LOOKING BACK

### A. Mercury Toxicity

1. Mercury exposure can occur through air, water, food and dental amalgams.
2. Safe levels of air mercury as indicated by OSHA are reliable neither for dental patients nor dental staff.
3. There are factors other than a recent exposure to mercury that influence the levels of mercury in blood, urine and hair.
4. Toxic mercury levels on a group basis are more reliable than on an individual basis.
5. On an individual basis, blood mercury is the most reliable test for exposure to mercury.
6. Mercury can be distributed in any of its three forms.
7. Adverse effects may include inflammation, interference with sulfhydryl and disulfide groups and therefore, with amino acids, enzymes and ligands. These interferences can occur in many biological systems.

### B. Mercury Allergy

1. Allergy to mercury is one of the most common causes of allergic dermatitis.
2. Sensitivity is latent in healthy and non-allergic individuals.
3. Sensitivity is manifested locally and systemically.
4. There is usually a non-dental sensitizing experience in the patient's history.
5. Patch testing is useful if hypersensitivity is suspected but is not known.

# REFERENCES

1. "Dentists, Staff Members Healthy, Despite Daily Contact with Mercury," *ADA News* (Chicago), December 1983.
2. "Recommendations in Dental Mercury Hygiene, 1984," Council on Dental Materials, Instruments, and Equipment, *JADA*, Vol. 109, October 1984.
3. "Safety of Dental Amalgam," Council on Dental Materials, Instruments and Equipment and Council of Dental Therapeutics, *JADA*, vol. 106, April 1983.
4. Reinhardt, J., Boyer, D., Svare, C., Frank, C., Cox, R. and Gay, D.: "Exhaled Mercury Following Removal and Insertion of Amalgam Restorations," *J Prosthet Dent*, 49(5):652–656, 1983.
5. Bauer, J. and First, H.: "The Toxicity of Mercury in Dental Amalgam," *CDA Journal*, 10:47–61, June 1982.
6. Utt, H.: "Mercury Breath . . . How much is too much?" *CDA Journal*, 12(2):41–45, February 1984.
7. Cooley, R. and Young, J.: "Detection and Diagnosis of Bioincompatibility of Mercury," *CDA Journal*, 12(10):36–43, October 1984.
8. Anusavice, K., Soderholm, K., Mohammed, H., and Shen, C.: "Consequences of Mercury Exposure in Dentistry: A Review of the Literature," *Fla Dent J*, 54(4):17–19, Winter 1983.
9. Leirskar, J.: "On the Mechanisms of Cytotoxicity of Silver and Copper Amalgams in a Cell System," *Scand J Dent Res*, 82(1):74–81, 1974.
10. Frykholm, K.: "On Mercury from Dental Amalgam, Its Toxic and Allergic Effects and Some Comments on Occupational Hygiene," *Acta Odont Scand*, 15(suppl 22):1–108, 1957.
11. Svare, C., Frank, C. and Chan, K.: "Quantitative Measure of Mercury Vapor Emission from Settling Dental Amalgam," *J Dent Res*, 52:740–743, July–Aug, 1973.
12. Svare, C.: "Dental Amalgam Related Mercury Vapor Exposure," *CDA Journal*, 17(10):54–58, October, 1984.
13. Chan, K. and Svare, C.: "Mercury Vapor Emission from Dental Amalgam," *J Dent Res*, pp. 555–559, March–April 1972.
14. Svare, C., Peterson, L., Reinhardt, J., Frank, C. and Boyer, D.: "Dental Amalgam: A Potential Source of Mercury Vapor Exposure," *J of Dent Res*, 59 (Special Issue A):391, Abstract #293, March 1980.
15. Svare, C., Peterson, L., Reinhardt, J., Boyer, D., Frank, C., Gay, D. and Cox, R.: "The Effects of Dental Amalgams on Mercury levels in Expired Air," *J Dent Res*, 60(9):1668–1671, September, 1981.
16. Freden, H., Hellden, L. and Milledig, P.: "Mercury Content in Gingival Tissues Adjacent to Amalgam Fillings," *Odonto Rev*, 25(2):207–210, 1974.
17. Hursh, J., Clarkson, T., Cherian, M., Vostal, J. and Vander Malie, R.: "Clearance of Mercury Vapor Inhaled by Human Subjects," *Arch Environ Health*, 31:302–309, 1976.
18. Moller, B.: "Reactions of Human Dental Pulp to Silver Amalgam Restorations, Mercury Determination in Dental Pulps by Flameless Atomic Absorption Spectrophotometry," *Swed Dent J*, 2:93–97, 1978.

19. Holland, G. and Asgar, K.: "Some Effects on the Phases of Amalgam Induced by Corrosion," *J Dent Res*, 53:1245–1254, 1974.
20. Chan, S.: "Amalgam Tattos (Localized Argyria): Review of the Literature," *Georgetown Dent J*, 42(2):34, July 1978.
21. Gay, D., Cox, R. and Reinhardt, J.: "Chewing Releases Mercury from Fillings," *Lancet* (letter) 1:985–986, May 5, 1979.
22. Stofen, D.: "Dental Amalgam—a Poison in Our Mouth," *Toxicology*, 2(4):355–358, December, 1974.
23. Radics, J., Schwander, H. and Gasser, F.: "Die Kristallinin Komponenten Der Silberamalgam Untersuchungen, mit der Electronischen Röntgenmikrosorde," *Zahnarztl Welt*, 79:1031–1036, 1970.
24. Goldwater, L., Ladd, A. and Jacobs, M.: "Absorption and Excretion of Mercury in Man," *Arch Environmental Health*, 9:6, 1964.
25. Hensten-Pettersen, A.: "Metabolism of Degradation/Corrosion Products from Tissue–Material Interactions," *Biomaterials* 5:42–46, January 1984.
26. Heintze, U., Edwardson, S., Derand, T. and Birkhed, D.: "Methylation of Mercury from Dental Amalgam and Mercuric Chloride by Oral Streptococci in Vitro," *Scand J Dent Res*, 91(2):150–152, April 1983.
27. Greener, E.: "Amalgam—Yesterday, Today and Tomorrow," *Oper Dent*, 4(1):24–35, Winter 1979.
28. Rowland, I., Grasso, P. and Davies, M.: "The Methylation of Mercuric Chloride by Human Intestinal Bacteria," *Experientia* 31:1064, 1975.
29. Gabuten, G., Persona. Communication, FDA, Rockville, Md., March 22, 1985.
30. Hidemitsu, S., Pan-Hou, H., Hosono, M. and Imura, N.: "Plasmid-Controlled Mercury Biotransformation by Clostridium Cochlearium T-2," *Applied Environ Micro*, 40(6):1007–1011, December 1980.
31. Goldwater, L.: "The Toxicology of Inorganic Mercury," *Annals of NY Acad Sci*, 65(5):498–503, April 1957.
32. Gilman, A., Goodman, L. and Gilman, A.: *The Pharmacological Basis of Therapeutics*, Macmillan Pub. Co., New York, 1980.
33. Kawahara, H., Nakamura, H., Yamagami, A., and Nakanishi, T.: "Cellular Response to Dental Amalgam in Vitro," *J Dent Res*, 54(2):394–401, March–April, 1975.
34. Rupp, N, and Paffenbarger, J.: "Significance to Health of Mercury Used in Dental Practice: A Review," *J Amer Dent Assoc*, 82(6): 1401–1407, June 1971.
35. Clarkson, T., Gatzy, J. and Dalton, C.: "Studies on the Equilibration of Mercury Vapor with Blood," U of Rochester Atomic Energy Project, January 1961.
36. Kuntz, W., Pitkin, R., Bostrum, A. and Hughes, M.: "Maternal and Cord Blood Background Mercury Levels: A Longitudinal Surveillance," *Am J Obstet Gynecol*, 143:440–443, 1982.
37. Glickman, I. and Imber, I.: "Comparison of Gingival Resection with Electrosurgery and Peridontal Knives—A Biometric and Histological Study," *J Perio*, 41:142–148, 1970.

38. Hurt, W., Nabors, C. and Rose, G.: "Some Clinical and Histological Observation of Gingiva Treated by Cryotherapy," *J Periodontol*, 43:151–156, 1972.
39. Loe, H.: "Chemical Gingivectomy—Effect of Potassium Hydroxide on Peridontal Tissue," *Acta Odont Scand*, 19:517–535, 1961.
40. Goldschmidt, P., Cogen, R. and Taubman, S.: "Effects of Amalgam Corrosion Products on Human Cells," *J Perio Res*, 11:108–115, 1976.
41. Souder, W. and Sweeney, W.: "Is Mercury Poisonous in Dental Amalgam Restorations?" *Dent Cosmos*, LXXXII(12):1145–1152, December, 1931.
42. Vallee, B. and Ulmer, D.: "Biochemical Effects of Mercury, Cadmium and Lead," *Ann Rev Biochem*, 44:91–128, 1972.
43. Chambers, J., Christoph, G., Krieger, M., Kay, L. and Stroud, R.: "Silver Ion Inhibition of Service Proteases: Crystallagraphic Study of Silvertrypsin," *Biochem and Biphysics Res Comm*, 59:70–74, 1974.
44. Hughes, W.: "A Physiochemical Rationale for the Biological Activity of Mercury and its Compounds," *Annals of NY Acad Sci*, 65(5):454–460, April 1957.
45. Abraham, J., Svare, C. and Frank, C.: "The Effects of Dental Amalgam Restorations on Blood Mercury Levels," *J Dent Res*, 63(1):71–73, 1984.
46. Schopf, E., Schultz, K. and Isensee, I.: "Untersuchunger wenn den lymphocytentraus formations-Test bei Quicksilber-Allergie," *Arch Klin Exp Derm*, 234:420–433, 1969.
47. Djerassi, E. and Berova, N.: "The Possibilities of Allergic Reactions from Silver Amalgam Restorations," *Int Dent J*, 19(4):481–488, December 1969.
48. Duxbury, A., Ead, R., McMurrough, S. and Watts, D.: "Allergy to Mercury in Dental Amalgam," *Br Dent J*, 152:47–48, January 1982.
49. Duxbury, A., Watts, D. and Ead, R.: "Allergy to Dental Amalgam," *Br Dent J*, 152:344–345, May 18, 1982.
50. Fernstrom, A., Frykholm, K., and Huldt, S.: "Mercury Allergy with Eczematous Dermatitis Due to Silver Amalgam Fillings," *Br Dent J*, 113:204–206, September 1962.
51. Shoveton, D.: "Silver Amalgam and Mercury Allergy," *Oral Surg*, 25(1):29–30, January, 1968.
52. Spector, L.: "Allergic Manifestations to Mercury," *J Amer Dent Assoc*, 42:320, 1951.
53. Thomson, J. and Russell, J.: "Dermatitis Due to Mercury Following Amalgam Dental Restorations," *Br J Derm*, 82(3):292–297, 1970.
54. White, I. and Smith, B.: "Dental Amalgam Dermatitis," *Br Dent J*, 156(7):259–260, 1984.
55. Engleman, M.: "Mercury Allergy Resulting From Amalgam Restorations," *J Amer Dent Assoc*, 66:122–123, January 1963.
56. Soremark, R., Ingels, O., Platt, H. and Smsahl, K.: "Influences of Some Dental Restorations of the Concentration of Inorganic Constitutents of the Teeth," *Acta Odont Scand*, 20:215–224, 1962.

57. Lawrence, D.: "Heavy Metals Modulation of Lymphocyte Activities," *Toxicology and Applied Pharm*, 57:439–451.
58. Arnold, N.: "Allergy to Mercury in Amalgam Fillings," (letter), *J Amer Med Assoc*, Queries and Minor Notes, 111:646, August 1983.
59. Fuerman, E.: "Recurrent Contact Dermatitis Caused by Mercury in Amalgam Dental Fillings," *Intern'l J Dermatol*, 14(9):657–660, November 1975.
60. Ellender, G., Ham, K. and Harcourt, J.: "Toxic Effects of Dental Amalgam Implants, Optical, Histological, and Histochemical Observation," *Aust Dent J*, 23(5):395–399, October 1978.
61. Catsakis, L. and Sulica, V.: "Allergy to Silver Amalgams," *Oral Surg*, 46(3):371–375, September 1978.
62. Eggleston, D.: "Effect of Dental Amalgam and Nickel Alloys of T-lymphocytes: Preliminary Report," *J Pros Dent*, 51(5):617–623, May 1984.
63. Fregert, S. and Bandman, H.: *Patch Testing*, Springer-Verlag, New York, p. 2, 1975.
64. Huggins, H.: "What is Mercury Toxicity?," Basic Information Packet, Colorado Springs, Colorado, 1984.
65. Huggins, H. and Huggins, S.: *It's All in Your Head*, Colorado Springs, Colorado, 1985.
66. "Patch tests for Sensitivity to Mercury or Nickel," Council on Dental Materials, Instruments and Equipment and Council on Dental Therapeutics, *JADA* 108:381, March 1984.
67. Ingalls, T.: "Epidemiology, Etiology, and Prevention of Multiple Sclerosis," *Amer J Forensic Med Path*, 4(1):55–60, March 1983.
68. Williams, R.: "Some Features of Antibiotic Resistance in Staphylococci: Mercury Resistance and Multiple Antibiotic Resistance," *Proc R Soc Med*, 64:540, 1971.
69. Finne, K., Goransson, K. and Winckler, L.: "Oral Lichen Planus and Contact Allergy to Mercury," *Int J Oral Surg*, 11:236–239, August 1982.
70. Lundstrom, I.: "Allergy and Corrosion of Dental Materials in Patients with Oral Lichen Planus," *Int J Oral Surg*, 13:16–24, February 1984.
71. Markow, H.: "Urticaria Following a Dental Silver Filling-Case Report," *NY St J Med*, 43:1648–1652, 1943.
72. Ganong, W.: *Review of Medical Physiology*, Lange Med Pub, Los Altos, California, pp. 414–421, 1983.
73. Pleva, J.: "Mercury Poisoning From Dental Amalgam," *Orthomolecular Psychiatry*, 12(3):184–193, 1983.

# 9
# PUTTING
# IT
# TOGETHER

LOOKING AHEAD

1. THINGS THAT CAN HELP OR HURT US
   A. Overview
   B. Mental Attitude
   C. Nutrition
   D. Exercise
   E. Rest, Relaxation and Biofeedback
   F. Love
   G. Laughter
2. THINGS THAT CAN *ONLY* HURT US
   A. Overview
   B. Lifestyle
   C. Chemicals Used in the Workplace
   D. Chemicals Used in the Home
   E. Toxic Heavy Metals
3. DENTAL AMALGAMS AS A SOURCE OF MERCURY EXPOSURE
   A. Overview
   B. The Use of Mercury in Dentistry
   C. The Amalgam Filling
   D. The Biotransformation of Mercury
   E. The Distribution of Mercury
   F. Mercury Toxicity
   G. Mercury Allergy
4. DISEASES RELATED TO MERCURY EXPOSURE

LOOKING BACK

## LOOKING AHEAD

Health is the ingredient that separates merely being alive from fully enjoying life. In our search for optimum health, we find things that are a help and other things that are a hindrance in our journey. Along our paths we must evaluate ourselves and our environment. Things that are good for us go on one side of our health scale; things that hurt us go on the other side.

In this chapter, we will examine where dental amalgam fillings fit into the total picture and you will learn how to tip the scale in your favor.

## 1. THINGS THAT CAN HELP OR HURT US

### A. Overview

In chapter one, we saw that a simple vitamin can help us if we take only what we need; that same vitamin can hurt us if we take too much. Like vitamins, other things can help us or hurt us. Some of these things include our mental attitude; our nutrition; our exercise program; our concept of and participation in rest, relaxation and biofeedback; the existence of love in our lives and our ability to laugh. Let's look at each factor individually.

### B. Mental Attitude

The first step we must take on our journey towards optimal health is to know what level of health we want. If our expectations are high, we will not be satisfied with relieving symptoms with a pill. We must work with our health professionals to identify and alleviate factors in our environment that predispose us to disease. Prevention will be our top priority. With the advice of our physicians, we must decide on our health plan; we must say YES to the things that help us and NO to the things that hurt us.

### C. Nutrition

Number one on the "help" side of our health scale is nutrition. We have seen that the better the quality of our supply of nutrients, the better able we are to stay healthy. Water and air can go on either side of our scale depending on whether they are free from contaminants. If the water is pure and the air is pollution-free, they are on the help side of the scale because they are essential ingredients for life.

Food also can go on either side of the scale depending on *who gets to it before it gets to you*. I remember attending a vitamin and nutrition seminar given by Dr. Emanuel Cheraskin. Among the important things that I learned that day was Dr. Cheraskin's comments on food. He said: ". . . if man touched it, don't eat it!" Basically what he was saying was that whole, unprocessed, unadulterated food is best for us.

The most nutritious way of eating is to have a great variety of fresh fruit, fresh vegetables, whole grains and an assortment of legumes and meat to satisfy our protein requirements. Clinical ecologists (physicians who specialize in environmental medicine) routinely recommend a Rotary Diversified Diet to allergy patients.[1–5] This Rotary Diversified Diet was developed by Dr. Rinkel[5] for food-allergic patients. This diet enables allergy patients to identify foods to which they are allergic and allows those patients to avoid developing new food allergies. Patients cannot eat a particular food more often than once in four days with a 48-hour separation between foods of the same family (e.g., beef and lamb).

There are things that can be done to good, nutritious food which will put it on the "hurt" side of the scale. The food itself can hurt us if it produces allergic symptoms and we continue to eat it. In addition, food can be put on the hurt side of the scale long before it gets to us. Some farmers use soil additives, chemical fertilizers, pesticides or herbicides which are toxins and, as such, add to the total toxic load of our bodies. The use of antibiotics in livestock can affect our own physiology. When we eat meat from these animals, we may alter the normal bacteria living in our intestines.

Food processing also can add substances which may be harmful to us. Examples of these substances are nitrates, nitrites, artificial coloring, artificial flavoring and preservatives. Some of the "staysoft" cookies stay soft because of added plastics!

Finally, the method we use to cook our food can put it on the hurt side of the scale. High heat can destroy some vitamins and can alter the fat of meats to create unhealthy compounds. Cooking in aluminum pots and pans can destroy certain vitamins; plastic coated pots can add chemicals to our food.

Of course, because we live in the twentieth century, it is difficult to find food that does not contain some pesticide residue. These things are "out of our control." It is important for us to be aware that we are getting toxins from the air we breath (industrial pollution), the water we drink (chemicals and other toxins) and the food we eat (pesticides, toxins and heavy metals). Sometimes we have to compromise on our ideals; but it is important to always avoid unnecessary exposure to chemicals and toxins.

Physiological defects, such as diabetes, may interfere with nutrition. These defects go on the hurt side of our scale because they create an imbalance in our bodies which impairs our bodily functions. Other examples of physiological defects are a lack of hydrochloric acid in our stomachs which interferes with digestion and low or faulty insulin production which can lead to excess sugar in the blood and which may result in eye damage, kidney damage or reduced healing. Some scientists believe that many metabolic disorders and physiological defects can be caused by toxins as well as by genetic abnormalities. If this belief is correct, a vicious cycle is in progress; toxins can cause physiological disturbances which in turn result in a decreased ability to handle additional toxins.

### D. Exercise

Everyone agrees that exercise is good for us. Exercise increases blood flow which efficiently distributes nutrients and carries off waste products and toxins. It strengthens our hearts and has a positive effect on our entire bodies. Because of this positive effect, exercise is on the help side of the scale.

### E. Rest, Relaxation and Biofeedback

Most of us consider rest to be what we do when we are too tired to work or play. Relaxation, on the other hand, involves a more active role whether we read, fish, golf or participate in some similar activity. Relaxation relieves the tension created by work or other stressful activities.

Biofeedback takes relaxation a step further. It is a deliberate action used to gain some voluntary control over our automatic (autonomic) body functions. Examples of automatic body function are blood pressure, temperature and pain. This biofeedback technique is based on the fact that a specific thought or action can produce a desired response (e.g., lower blood pressure). By practicing biofeedback or relaxation exercises, we can accomplish such things as lowering our blood pressure and ultimately alter the way we react to stresses. If we are able to reduce our stress reactions which use a up a lot of energy and nutrients, we can allow our bodies to function more efficiently.

Dr. Carl Simonton has taken biofeedback and added yet another dimension: that of imagery.[6] Imagery or visualization involves several steps: first, the patient uses a relaxation process. Second, the patient selects a desired goal to be achieved. Third, the patient paints, in his or her mind's eye, a picture having already accomplished that goal. Dr. Simonton introduced the concept of imagery (visualizing certain physiological events) to help patients in their healing process. Some allergy patients have used such visualization in attempting to stimulate their immune systems. As a part of a biofeedback or relaxation exercise, the patient visualizes "pac-man" shaped white blood cells chasing, catching and eating different toxins or infectious agents. Although visualization is controversial, it helps some patients. Because it helps patients, visualization goes on the help side of our scale.

### F. Love

Many of us take love for granted and don't realize its importance in staying healthy. Sidney Baker, M.D., Research Director of the Gesell Institute for Human Development (New Haven, Connecticut), has included love in his expanded concept of "nutrition." Dr. Baker indicates that love is an essential nutrient for our wellbeing. Because of the positive influence love has on our general wellbeing, it is put on the help side of the scale.

### G. Laughter

Our body chemistry is affected by positive and negative emotions. During illness, our negative emotions generally prevail. In order to enhance our body, Norman Cousins suggests a program for exercising our affirmative emotions.[7] Mr. Cousins suggests that:

> "[Laughter] provides exercise for [a] person . . . a form of jogging for the innards . . . [laughter] creates a mood in which the other positive emotions can be put to work. In short, [laughter] helps make it possible for good things to happen."[7]

## 2. THINGS THAT CAN *ONLY* HURT US

### A. Overview

In the last section, I discussed factors that could change something that is beneficial into something that is harmful. Whole wheat flour, for example, is very nutritious and can help you. If that same flour is processed to white flour, most of its nutritional value is removed. Food companies then attempt to make up for those lost nutrients by adding certain vitamins and minerals. This attempt is futile because they are not able to replace all the essential trace nutrients lost through processing. This same processing scenario is repeated in many foods.

Although the reasons (decreased cost and increased production) for using pesticides and herbicides are well intentioned, there are alternatives which are less costly in terms of our health. We end up paying the price one way or the other.

In this section, I will discuss some things that can *only* hurt you. These include alcohol, tobacco, caffeine, chemicals at home and in the workplace and dental mercury.

### B. Lifestyle

We may purchase nutritious foods and cook them properly; we may not have physiological abnormalities which increase our need for certain nutrients or decrease our ability to use those nutrients; but, we may still be doing something which compromises our nutritional status. What can we be doing wrong? We may have a counterproductive lifestyle. Such a lifestyle would include the use of alcoholic beverages, caffeine or tobacco.

Alcohol destroys vitamins A and B complex and interferes with the minerals potassium and zinc. Caffeine interferes with vitamins A and B complex and the minerals iron, potassium and zinc. Tobacco interferes with B1, B2, B6, B12, folic acid, C, and bioflavonoids. Taking drugs and medications (even prescription) add to our lifestyle stresses by interfering with our nutritional status. An example of this is in the use of oral contraceptives. These interfere with B vitamins, vitamin C and vitamin D as well as the minerals copper, magnesium and zinc.

If our daily routine includes stress at home or stress at the office, our nutritional status may also be compromised. Stress destroys B complex vitamins and vitamin C and interferes with the minerals calcium and potassium.

### C. Chemicals Used in the Workplace

The chemicals in our lives may do considerable harm to us. Chemicals used in industry can be toxic and interfere with bodily processes as discussed in Chapter One, Physiology, and Chapter Two, Toxicity. Of course, many of us cannot leave our jobs. Alternative work situations may be as harmful as our present jobs. What we must do is minimize our exposures to toxins by following the guidelines set out by the manufacturers of those materials we use at work and by using common sense. The cleanest air and the best environment may be found high on a deserted mountain; but, without work and without social interactions, we may be no better off than we are in our present environment. We need goals, we need communication and we need stimulation in order to survive.

### D. Chemicals Used in the Home

The chemicals we use in and around our homes are "under our control." We might ask ourselves: Do we need a greener lawn than our neighbors? Are we willing to have chemicals sprayed on our lawns at the risk of exposing ourselves to toxins every time we open the windows or sit in the backyard?

I want to mention briefly some of the chemicals we use daily to give you a general concept of the chemical-toxin problem. These chemicals are in addition to the additives, pesticides and preservatives found in our food and water. Many of these chemicals put a physiological stress on our systems; but, not knowing this, we continue to use them. We wake up in the morning on our no-iron sheets—formaldehyde makes them permanent-press. These sheets may contain polyester which is a petrochemical. The detergent which we used to wash the sheets contains many caustic agents and petrochemicals (including perfume) any of which can have a toxic effect. In addition to the detergent, our fabric softener contains more chemicals and perfume to hide the smell of these chemicals. We were breathing in these chemicals all night. When we get up in the morning, our first stop is the shower. If we use city water, it contains chlorine which we breath in as the hot water vaporizes. Our deodorant soap contains so many ingredients, I can't list them here. Ditto for the shaving cream. After shave lotion or perfume is an interesting toxin by itself. It is absorbed through the skin and is circulated throughout the body until your liver can detoxify it. This exposure takes place over a 24-hour period. Our toothpaste also contains synthetic colorings, flavorings, preservatives and a variety of other ingredients. I can go on forever!

These home chemicals are under our control. There are many books available which can help you identify the chemicals and toxins in your life. They will also tell you what alternatives are available for cleaning, washing and for personal hygiene (see Suggested Reading).

### E. Toxic Heavy Metals

Heavy metals are toxic for three reasons: first, they cannot be broken down by our bodies; second, they accumulate in various cells and tissues; and third, they combine with one or more compounds which may have important physiological function. There are three heavy metals which we should be concerned about: lead, mercury and cadmium. Lead and mercury produce very similar symptoms. I might mention that at a concentration level that causes problems, most toxins cause symptoms that are similar and, in most cases, the toxin cannot be identified by the patient's symptoms. Exposure to these heavy metals can occur from the air we breathe, the water we drink, and the food we eat. This exposure is cumulative; that is, we must examine *all* sources of exposure (food, water, dental fillings, etc.) in order to determine our toxic load. If your goal is to eliminate all mercury from your environment, you may want to completely avoid seafood, which is known to contain mercury compounds.

## 3. DENTAL AMALGAM AS A SOURCE OF MERCURY EXPOSURE

### A. Overview

Dental amalgam fillings are a source of mercury exposure. In this section I will discuss what happens once you leave the dental office with an amalgam filling in your tooth. I've selected a question-and-answer format because I believe this approach will answer some of the many questions you have about dental mercury and health.

### B. The Use of Mercury in Dentistry

1) *How extensively is mercury used in dentistry?*

Approximately 75 percent of all dental fillings are dental amalgam.

2) *How much mercury is in dental amalgam?*

Dental amalgam fillings contain about 50 percent mercury when placed in your mouth.

3) *How is mercury used in dentistry?*

Mercury has three applications in dentistry. All three use amalgam. First, mercury is used in amalgam fillings; second, dental amalgam is used to build up a tooth that has had either a lot of decay or needs additional support in order to be crowned (capped); and third, dental amalgam is sometimes used to seal the root-tip of a tooth which is undergoing root canal therapy. I want to clarify this last application of amalgam which is sometimes performed on front teeth (see Figure 3). As part of root canal treatment, access to the root of the tooth is gained by cutting the gum adjacent to the bone covering the root-tip. At this point, an opening is made in the bone.

The root-tip is then prepared for an amalgam filling (called a retrograde amalgam). The amalgam filling is placed in the root-tip in order to seal the root canal. The opening is closed and allowed to heal. Although this amalgam filling is placed in the root-tip, the root-tip is within the bone. In light of the information contained in the literature, this procedure should be avoided.

*Figure 3:* **Retrograde Amalgam**

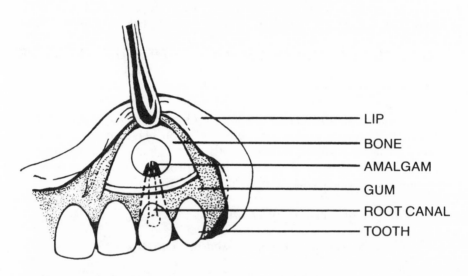

LIP
BONE
AMALGAM
GUM
ROOT CANAL
TOOTH

### C. The Amalgam Filling

1) *Is mercury given off by amalgam fillings?*

Once the amalgam filling is placed, it continually liberates mercury vapor. This liberation occurs because of corrosion and wear. The presence of other metals in the mouth, such as gold crowns (caps) and metal partial dentures, *accelerates* the release of mercury vapor. Chewing also causes the release of mercury vapor. It has been suggested that we are exposed to mercury vapor from fillings during gestation (from our mother's amalgam fillings) and afterwards from our own amalgam fillings.

2) *How much mercury vapor is liberated by the amalgam filling?*

Scientists have estimated that as much as 25 to 45 ug of mercury per day could be liberated by amalgam fillings. The amount liberated depends on the type of alloy used for the filling, the amount of mercury contained in the amalgam filling when it is placed, the presence of other metals in the mouth and the amount of chewing.

3) *How much mercury vapor is needed to cause a problem for patients?*

If we are looking for the minimum amount of mercury vapor which can cause a problem, then this is a difficult question to answer. It is difficult to answer because there are several factors to evaluate. Among these factors are the period of exposure, the number of different sources of mercury, the individual's susceptability and the additive effects of other toxins.

First, there is a lot of information on the effects of an acute, high-dose exposure to mercury. There is less information on the chronic, low-dose exposure to mercury. People who have amalgam fillings have a chronic, low-dose exposure. The question we have to answer is whether this low dose is high enough to cause a problem over a period of time. The literature does not contain information about the minimum amount of mercury exposure necessary to interfere with biological systems. The literature describes a laboratory experiment where a "small" amount of mercuric ion was sufficient for cellular damage to occur and that only $10^{-4}$ to $10^{-6}$ molar concentration (molar concentration is the standard concentration of a substance in a liter of solution) was enough to cause the inhibition of amino acid incorporation into protein-like substances in cell culture. In this case, a dilution of one ten-thousandth (1/10,000) to one millionth (1/1,000,000) could interfere with the formation of "protein" from amino acids. You can see that damage can occur with very small doses of mercury.

Second, mercury accumulates in your body. Therefore, if you are exposed to mercury from several sources, a lower amount of mercury from each source will be sufficient to cause harm. For example, if you eat large amounts of fish (tuna, shellfish, swordfish, salmon, cod, pike and perch), the mercury contained in those fish adds to your total body burden of mercury.

Third, your individual susceptibility is an important factor. Both genetic weaknesses and an inability to detoxify mercury lowers the amount of mercury needed to cause a problem for you.

Fourth, the additive effects of toxins are related to your body's overall ability to detoxify itself. If you are exposed to several toxins at the same time, then it will be more difficult for your body to detoxify and excrete each toxin. Consequently, a lower dose of each toxin can cause symptoms. For example, the patient with candidiasis (infection of Candida albicans) is exposed to toxins which increase that patient's toxic load.

4) *How long a period of time are you exposed to the mercury that comes from your fillings?*

The half-time for all forms of mercury is approximately 65 days (in the brain, 18 to 22 years). This means that if 100 ug of mercury exist in your body initially, then there would be 50 ug remaining in your body after 65 days, assuming no additional exposure. However, amalgams liberate mercury vapor on a continuous basis because of corrosion and because of chewing. This mercury enters your body and is capable of interfering with biological activities. The extent of interference depends on the amount of mercury entering your body, your rate of detoxifying mercury and your rate of mercury excretion. A biologically efficient individual would have less interference from a toxin than would a biologically inefficient individual. A typical example of a patient who would have a greater inhalation of mercury from amalgam fillings is an asthmatic (or a patient with chronic sinusitis) with many corroded amalgam fillings who is on a restricted hypoglycemic diet (having to eat 6 small meals a day and, therefore, chewing approximately three hours a day).

5) *Where does the mercury go?*

The mercury vapor liberated by the dental amalgam filling can enter the body in four ways: it can enter the pulp, the adjacent soft tissues, the lungs and the GI tract. First, mercury vapor can be found in the dental pulp within 10 days after placement of an amalgam filling. Second, gingival tissues adjacent to amalgam fillings contain as much as 49 times as much mercury as in gingival tissues not adjacent to amalgam fillings. Third, mercury vapor released during chewing enters the lungs. Fourth, although not in the literature, we can assume that mercury vapor enters the GI tract since some of the air that we breath goes into our stomachs and there is the possibility of mercury attaching to some food materials during chewing.

**D. Biotransformation of mercury vapor to methyl mercury**

1) *Is mercury vapor converted to methyl mercury?*

There is evidence that mercury vapor is converted to methyl mercury by various microorganisms normally present in the mouth and GI tract. The experiments which demonstrate this were done in the laboratory. However, there is no evidence that these organisms biotransform mercury vapor into methyl mercury when they are in the body.

2) *Is methyl mercury biotransformed into mercury vapor?*

Methyl mercury is biotransformed to mercury vapor by the same strains (family) of microorganisms that convert mercury vapor to methyl mercury. This is also a laboratory experiment. There is also no evidence that these organisms biotransform methyl mercury into mercury vapor when they are in the body.

3) *What proof is there that mercury vapor is biotransformed into methyl mercury in the body?*

The only proof that mercury is converted to methyl mercury in the body is by indirect evidence; that is, because mercury is converted to methyl mercury in the laboratory, it is postulated that this reaction occurs in the body. However, we don't know for sure if mercury does undergo conversion in the human body.

### E. The Distribution of Mercury

1) *Once in your body, where does mercury go?*

Mercury vapor enters the blood and combines with various compounds. It is then distributed throughout the entire body. After some time, it accumulates in the tissues and organs containing the compounds with which it has the strongest attraction (nervous tissue) or in the organs of excretion (kidney and liver).

2) *How long does mercury stay in the body?*

The half-time for mercury is approximately 65 days. This figure can rise to 18 to 22 years for mercury contained in the brain.

### F. Mercury Toxicity

1) *Is the mercury that comes out of the amalgam fillings toxic?*

The answer is a qualified yes. If the mercury ion attaches to a compound (e.g., an enzyme), it will alter the function of that compound. In the case of an enzyme, mercury would be toxic to that enzyme system. *If* you are able to rapidly remove that mercury ion from that enzyme and excrete it, it is no longer toxic. As you can see, toxicity depends on the substance *and* the susceptibility of the individual.

2) *What are some of the biological effects mercury can have on our bodies?*

Mercury is chemically attracted to sulfur, nitrogen, oxygen and the halogens. Because of this attraction, mercury has the potential to cause adverse reactions by attaching to various minerals and compounds such as amino acids and proteins (hemoglobin and enzymes). The resulting complex (mercury and the compound in the body) may alter the action of these compounds and may result in decreased efficiency or impairment of function in the mercury-exposed patient. Which biological systems can be affected will vary with the individual's genetic weaknesses and the doses of mercury exposure. Remember that acute mercury toxicity results in disturbances in the neurological system (motor coordination, emotional symptoms, personality disturbances and headache), the GI tract (diarrhea, nausea and loss of appetite), kidney and the immune system. Sub-acute toxicity (between acute and chronic) may result in sub-clinical impairment (no signs or symptoms). This last bit of information is important because we can be on the road to disease without knowing it. It is also important to understand that if you have a high amount of other toxins in your environment, mercury will have a greater effect because your body may be overburdened in its attempt to detoxify itself.

3) *What are the symptoms of micromercurialism (chronic low-dose exposure)?*

As you saw in Chapter Four, "Mercury," Trakhtenberg[8] relates symptoms of chronic low-dose exposure to mercury, first described by Stock,[9] as falling into three groups according to degree of intensity of the exposure:

> First-degree micromercurialism results in lowered working capacity, increased fatigue, light nervous excitability . . . in the second degree there is swelling of the nasal membranes, progressive weakening of memory, feelings of fear and loss of self-confidence, irritability, headaches. Simultaneously there may be catarrhal symptoms and upper respiratory discomfort, changes in the mucous membranes of the mouth, bleeding

gums. Sometimes there are feelings of coronary insufficiency, shivering, quickening pulse, and a tendency towards diarrhea. The third degree micromercurialism is characterized by symptoms approaching those of regular mercurialism [acute mercury exposure], but to a lesser degree. The symptoms of this stage are: headaches, general weakness, sleeplessness, decline in intellectual capacity, depression. Among other signs are tears, diarrhea, frequent urination, a feeling of pressure in the cardiac region and shivering.

4) *Who should be worried about mercury toxicity?*

Everyone should be concerned about the toxic effect of substances in their environment and should avoid all unnecessary exposures. This avoidance may include the replacement of amalgam fillings.

### G. Mercury Allergy

1) *Can we be allergic to the mercury in our amalgam fillings?*

We can be allergic to most of the metals (mercury, silver, tin or copper) used in dental amalgam as well as other metals (chromium, cobalt, nickel, palladium, and platinum) used in dentistry. Mercury by itself does not have the ability to produce an allergic response because it has a low molecular weight, but it does have the ability to combine (conjugate) with protein having sufficient molecular weight and cause an allergic response.

2) *Is there enough mercury liberated from amalgam fillings to cause an allergic reaction?*

Yes. The allergic response to an antigen depends on the concentration of that antigen. The literature is split on whether or not there is sufficient concentration of mercury liberated from amalgam fillings to support an allergic response. Supporting the belief that there is enough mercury are three pieces of evidence. First, the average patient can liberate 50 to 150 ug/m$^3$ of mercury from amalgam fillings after chewing for 10 minutes. Second, gingival tissue adjacent to amalgam fillings contained 49 times the mercury concentration (147 ug vs. 3.0 ug) than that of gingival tissue not adjacent to amalgam fillings. Third, Dr. John Santilli (Allergy Associates, Bridgeport, Connecticut) is able to stimulate the immune system with an antigen concentration in the range of $10^{-32}$ to $10^{-100}$. To further understand the concentration of Dr. Santilli's antigen solution, the number $1 \times 10^{-2}$

means the dilution is one one-hundredth the concentration (1/100th), $1 \times 10^{-3}$ is one one-thousandth (1/1,000th) the concentration. Picture the concentration of the highest of Dr. Santilli's solutions as having 32 zeros in all. That is 1/100,000,000,000,000,000,000,000,000, 000,000,000.

3) *What types of allergic reactions are caused by mercury?*

Both local and systemic allergic reactions to mercury have been reported in the literature. Published data and case studies indicate that dermatitis (a local reaction) and erythema (a systemic reaction) is sometimes caused by the placement or removal of an amalgam filling in mercury-sensitive patients.

4) *Is there truth to the statement that amalgam allergies will go away after the filling gets hard?*

When I first started to research mercury for this book, one of the first literature reviews I read was by Drs. Bauer and First.[10] In this article, Drs. Bauer and First stated that the course and the symptoms of mercury allergy were "self-limiting." I knew from previous reading about allergies that this was not so. In another literature review, Anusavice[11] quotes Wright[12] in indicating that allergic responses due to amalgam were "self-healing." However, in reviewing Wright's article, I didn't find any reference to self-healing or self-limiting. I am assuming that the authors (Drs. Bauer, First and Anusavice) believe that the allergy symptoms would go away when the amalgam completely hardened because researchers once thought that when amalgam hardened, no mercury could leave the filling and, therefore, an allergic reaction could no longer take place.

Randolph describes an alternative mechanism to allergy[1]. Dr. Randolph believes that an adapted stage results following the initial acute reaction to an allergen. In this stage there is a suppression of reactive symptoms. The second stage is followed by a maladapted stage and later by a nonadapted stage. Might this later stage be described as "latent?" In the maladapted stage, symptoms usually occur without any apparent relationship to the acute reaction. A possible mechanism operating in this case may be an alteration of the immune response and/or the production of an inflammatory response.

5) *How can you tell if you are allergic to mercury?*

There are two pieces of information to help you determine if you are allergic to mercury: your medical history and a mercury patch test. If you have a history of sensitivity to mercury-containing compounds (such as contraceptive jellies, eye ointment, merbromin, merthiolate, diuretics, contact lens solutions), or if you have a history of reactions to mercury you used in your school chemistry laboratory, or if you have had various unexplained reactions around the time you were having dental treatment done (amalgam fillings), you may suspect mercury sensitivity. The second piece of information you will need is the result of a mercury patch test. As you have seen, a mercury patch test indicates if a person is sensitive to mercury.

6) *Does the mercury from dental fillings affect the immune system?*

If the mercury from dental amalgams interferes with the immune system, amalgam fillings are a more serious health hazard than if it *only* causes local allergic reactions such as dermatitis. The implication that mercury has the potential to interfere with the immune system is extremely important because our very survival depends on our immune system. Dr. Eggleston's preliminary study tends to indicate that there is some effect on the immune system when either mercury or nickel is used as a filling material. The effect was to alter the quantity of T-cells. The mechanism of interfering with the immune system appears to be toxic rather than allergic. A more in-depth study is indicated to determine the effect that the mercury in dental amalgams would have on the number and function of the various subgroups of T-cells (T-helper, T-suppressor and T-effector cells). Potential reactions of mercury consist of attaching to cellular receptors, disulfide groups and sulfhydryl groups within the cells of the immune system. This attachment may result in a reduced ability by your body to recognize "self" or "foreign" protein, a reduced ability to manufacture antibodies or the impairment of vital toxin neutralization mechanisms.

7) *Can you be allergic to other dental materials?*

Patients can have allergic reactions to most of the dental chemicals and dental materials found in the dental office. An evaluation of the alternative filling materials is important if you have a tendency towards allergy. I have outlined the allergic potential of dental materials in another publication (see Suggested Readings).

8) *Does the acutely allergic patient have to be more careful about dental treatment?*

People have a wide range of responses to environmental substances. This range includes, for instance, the individual who has only experienced poison ivy and is not considered allergic, to those individuals who react to virtually everything with which they come into contact ("universal reactors"). I believe these differences in reaction are questions of degree. The individual reacting to poison ivy is displaying a maladaptive reaction to one substance. The environmentally ill universal reactor, in reacting to almost everything contacted, is displaying a maladapted reaction to many things. This is, in reality, an immune mechanism out of control. If mercury affected the operations of T-cells severely enough, can it too contribute to this loss of control?

*9) What is environmental illness?*

Environmental illness is a disease characterized by exaggerated responses to normal substances in your environment. The environmentally ill (EI) patients react to many substances in their environment. At this time it is not known exactly which of these reactions are true allergies and which are toxic reactions. What is known is that these individuals exhibit sensitivities to most of the following at some point in their illness:

1. Simple chemicals: formaldehyde, alcohol, chlorine, ammonia, bleach.
2. Petrochemicals: natural gas, gasoline, fuel oil, lubricating oil, perfumes, hair spray, moth balls, paint, plastics, solvents, pesticides.
3. Synthetics: permanent press (formaldehyde) and polyester clothing and plastics.
4. Smoke from wood or cooking.
5. Normal foods, food additives and growth stimulants existing in commercial meat.
6. Seasonal factors: pollen, grass, weeds, molds.
7. Building materials: these are combinations of chemicals and synthetics.
8. Vitamins: some are a combination of chemicals and foods.
9. Infectious agents: Candida albicans.
10. Metabolic dysfunction: inability to utilize nutrients properly.

EI patients exhibit these reactions from probably two mechanisms: toxic and allergic. They may react this way because their immune system is out of control (reacting to normal things in the environment) and that they have a decreased ability to detoxify or clear (excrete) certain chemicals in their environment or certain waste products of their own metabolism. Decreased clearance exists possibly because of decreased assimilation or faulty metabolism of nutrients. There is no certainty as to which comes first, the metabolic dysfunction or the disease.

Whatever the mechanisms operating in EI it is essential to deal with all factors playing a role in the disease, i.e. the diagnosis of offending substances, the avoidance of offending substances, Rotary Diversified Diet to minimize food reactions, nutritional support (vitamins, minerals, amino acids and fatty acids), immunotherapy (dust, molds and seasonals) and digestive support.

There are two points worth discussing; nutritional support and immunotherapy, which will give additional light to the "total load" with which EI patients must contend. EI patients appear to do better if their "load" is minimized. The load is simply the amount of exposure occurring in a given period of time. Balancing body chemistry, in vogue the past few years, consists of testing the patient for deficiencies of vitamins, minerals, amino acids and fatty acids and recommending supplements to replace those needed nutrients. Some clinical ecologists have suggested that the most productive supplementation program for EI patients, whose balance can be thrown off very easily, is to replace *only* those nutrients exhibiting a deficiency. For example, physicians have indicated that a deficiency in vitamin B6 is best treated with B6 rather than B-complex.

The second point concerns the three methods of immunotherapy: the traditional method, the end-point titration and the ultra low-dose therapy (very low concentration of antigen). The last two methods are used in treating ecological illness and accomplish both neutralization of symptoms and stimulation of the immune system. If one method doesn't help, the other may.

If the EI patient has greater sensitivity or is more allergy prone than average, increased sensitivity or allergy to mercury could be expected. Allergy to mercury will add to the allergic burden existing in that patient.

If the EI patient has a less than average clearance ability for toxins, then mercury may add to the burden of detoxification.

## 4. SYSTEMIC DISEASES RELATED TO MERCURY EXPOSURE

Some researchers have suggested that a wide variety of diseases are related to the mercury exposure from amalgam fillings. Among these diseases are multiple sclerosis, lichen planus, angina, arthritis, lupus erythematosis and such immune disorders as allergies, mononucleosis, leukemia, Hodgkin's disease and cancer. Although a few symptoms of some of these diseases may improve after amalgam replacement, you should not jump to the conclusion that the mercury from dental amalgam fillings is the cause of these diseases. Mercury is a toxin and, as such, puts a stress on our bodies. The removal of any toxin will reduce our total stress and would be expected to produce an improvement in the way we feel. I believe that it is highly probable that mercury contributes to neurological disorders and immune disorders and, as a result, may indirectly contribute to diseases related to these two systems. However, there is no scientific proof that mercury in amalgam fillings is the cause of any of these diseases; but, I believe that amalgam replacement should be considered as one of the tools used in treating systemic diseases involving the immune system.

## LOOKING BACK

1. You have seen that many factors contribute to health; other factors impair health.
2. There are some things which can help or hurt you depending on their purity.
3. There are some things which can only hurt you.
4. Dental amalgam falls on the hurt side of your health scale.

## REFERENCES

1. Randolph, T. and Moss, R.: *An Alternative Approach to Allergies*, Lippincott and Crowell, New York, pp. 69–83, 1979.
2. Crook, W.: *The Yeast Connection*, Professional Books, Jackson Tenn., pp. 9–14, 163–166, 1983.
3 . Dickey, L.: *Clinical Ecology*, Charles Thomas, Springfield, Ill., pp. 294–295, 1976.
4. Levin, A. and Dadd, D.: *A Consumer Guide for the Chemically Sensitive*, Alan Levin, San Francisco, pp. IX–XVIII, 1982.
5. Rinkel, H., Randolph, T. and Zeller, M.: *Food Allergy*, Charles C. Thomas, Springfield Ill., 1951.
6. Simonton, C., Matthews-Simonton, S. and Creighton, J.: *Getting Well Again*, Bantam Books, New York, 1978.
7. Cousins, N.: *Anatomy of an Illness*, Bantam Books, New York, p. 39, 1979.
8. Trakhtenberg, I.: *Chronic Effects of Mercury on Organisms* (Translation by Fogarty International Center for Advanced Study in the Health Sciences), U.S. Dept of HEW Public Service, National Institute of Health, D HEW Pub (NIH) 74–473, 1974.
9. Stock, A., *Z. Angew. Chem.*, 39:461, 1926.
10. Bauer, J. and First, H.: "The Toxicity of Mercury in Dental Amalgam," *CDA Journal*, 10:47–61, June 1982.
11. Anusavice, K., Soderholm, K., Mohammed, H, and Shen, C.: "Consequences of Mecury Exposure in Dentistry: A Review of the Literature," *Fla Dent J*, 54(4):17–19, Winter 1983.
12. Wright, F.: "Allergic Reaction to Mercury after Dental Treatment," *New Zealand Dent J*, 67(310):251–252, October, 1971.

# 10
# SURVEYS

LOOKING AHEAD

1. SURVEY OF CLINICAL ECOLOGISTS
   A. Letter
   B. Results of the Survey

2. SURVEY OF PATIENTS
   A. Publication and Letter
   B. Results of the Surveys

3. SURVEY OF DENTISTS
   A. Letter and Telephone Calls
   B. Results of the Surveys

4. EVALUATION OF THE SURVEYS

LOOKING BACK

## LOOKING AHEAD

In previous chapters, I discussed the two positions on dental mercury: the ADA position which maintains that dental mercury is safe and the anti-mercury position which maintains that dental mercury is poisonous. I also discussed the findings of scientists and researchers about the toxic potential of dental mercury and the effects that mercury may have on your health. This information is important in helping you to formulate an opinion about your own amalgam fillings.

To complete the picture, I have obtained feedback from clinical ecologists, patients and dentists; each of these groups has had direct experience with amalgam replacement. This clinical feedback is essential to evaluate the effects that mercury has had on the health of individuals who have already replaced their amalgam fillings. It also provides insight into what health improvements can be attributed to amalgam replacement. The full text of the surveys is in Appendix III.

AUTHOR'S NOTE: The information in this chapter was collected from answers received from surveys sent to clinical ecologists, patients and dentists. Improvements in health and alleviation of patients' symptoms described in this chapter are case histories. Advances in medicine have traditionally been made by "trial and error" with the individual practitioner observing improvement in his or her patient as a result of a specific treatment. More recently, science has become more sophisticated in that health professionals demand scientific proof that a particular set of circumstances resulted in the patient's improvement. These demands have led to "double-blind" studies where neither the subjects nor the experimenters know which prescribed drugs contain the active ingredient and which contain the placebo. An additional demand has been to revert the patient to the original circumstances to determine if those circumstances would again result in the patient's former illness. In the case of dental amalgam, the mercury-free fillings which replaced the amalgam fillings believed to be causing the patient's symptoms would again be replaced with amalgam to determine if the patient reverted back to the previous condition. Most practitioners would not suggest this to their patients just to prove a point especially in those patients who are acutely ill. Therefore, we must rely mostly on subjective information in the case of dental amalgam to indicate patient improvement until such a time that more measurable objective data are available.

# 1. SURVEY OF CLINICAL ECOLOGISTS

## A. Letter

I solicited help from clinical ecologists because their approach to medicine includes evaluation of many factors (especially environmental) involved in the disease process. As I discussed earlier, optimum health depends on such things as mental attitude, proper nutrition and your adaptation to your environment. Clinical ecologists routinely evaluate these factors. Because of their approach, I felt that the experience of clinical ecologists would provide objective information on the health consequences of dental mercury.

There are approximately 500 clinical ecologists who belong to the American Academy of Environmental Medicine. In January, 1985, I sent a survey to 20 clinical ecologists who I believed treated a sizable number of environmentally ill patients. The information that I requested included:

1) Whether the physician treated environmentally ill patients,
2) Whether a comprehensive examination and treatment plan was given to patients,
3) Whether dental amalgam replacement was part of their treatment plan,
4) Whether amalgam replacement took place,
5) At what point in the treatment was amalgam replacement done,
6) What dental materials were used to replace the amalgam fillings,
7) Whether the patient had any problems with the new fillings and
8) What role the physicians felt dental mercury played in environmental illness.

## B. Results of the survey

All clinical ecologists who responded to the survey did treat environmentally ill patients (those patients exhibiting symptoms of an allergy-sensitivity-metabolic-infection complex with acute sensitivity to environmental agents such as petrochemicals, foods, molds, seasonals, pollens and who are prone to infections such as Candida).

Their treatment plan included identification of the cause(s) of their patient's symptoms and a health plan which recommended elimination or avoidance of offending environmental substances, nutritional therapy, rotary diet, immune therapy, digestive therapy, prescription medications (to combat Candida infections) and amalgam replacement, when indicated.

The clinical ecologists responding to the survey indicated that when mercury is implicated in environmental disease, it is involved in two potential areas: toxicity and allergy. They also indicated that if mercury does play a role in environmental illness, it is but one of many factors. If a patient's history strongly suggests a link between dental mercury and their symptoms, the patient is referred to a dentist for a consultation. A patch test and electric current test are often performed by the dentist. A positive mercury sensitivity test results in a recommendation for amalgam replacement. The recommendation for mercury sensitivity testing was usually made towards the end of treatment. In some cases, the new filling material, usually gold or composite, was tested via skin tests. The type of replacement material most used was composite (white plastic filling material).

In response to the question which asked what role dental mercury plays in environmental illness, there was a wide range of responses by clinical ecologists. The most optimistic opinion concerning the health implications of dental mercury was that "Replacements [of dental amalgam fillings] have been remarkably successful . . . However, we are only replacing fillings where history and evaluation are positive . . . [dental mercury] plays a significant role in clinical ecology, but, it is certainly not the major factor."

It was suggested by another clinical ecologist that "Low grade heavy metal toxicity is certainly a real possibility and for many of the neurological difficulties that are found in these patients, I suspect that [dental] mercury has a significant impact."

Finally, another clinical ecologist suggested that, "With respect to environmental illness . . . I believe that EI patients will not get better until they remove their amalgam fillings."

On the other hand, one respondent indicated that:

> ". . . what I have been finding is largely poor results from removing dental amalgams . . . I sent four patients to have amalgams removed . . . three of these had no benefit, and one, a woman with scleroderma, had rather dramatic improvement in flexibility, appetite, energy and grip strength, all of which we had been monitoring beforehand. This improvement lasted approximately five weeks and was followed by a complete reversion to her previous symptom state and eventually her death." An additional nine patients with environmental illness ". . . have gone on their own to have amalgams removed . . .

one woman . . . had partial improvement in her headaches. Another . . . had improved . . . the other patients have all had no benefit whatsoever."

AUTHOR'S NOTE: The patients referred to in the first and the third opinions had used the sequential removal method for amalgam replacement. The last clinical ecologist further stated that "I think we do have to be very cautious about short-term evaluation of improvement in these patients."

Another clinical ecologist indicated a similar experience. He stated that:

"In my clinical experience, with a total of some six patients, I have seen no improvement in any one patient from the removal of the mercury amalgam . . . I have not been impressed by the results achieved by the removal of mercury amalgams and the use of supplements on the reduction of the levels of mercury in hair . . . I have achieved much better reduction [in the levels of hair mercury] in other patients by the use of selenium and by the use of nutritious diet under a well-controlled environmental program."

In general, in those cases where improvement did take place, the improvements noted as a result of amalgam replacement were increased energy level, increased appetite, better food and chemical tolerances and a decrease in the occurrence of headaches.

## 2. SURVEYS OF PATIENTS

### A. *Publications and letters*

Environmentally ill patients were surveyed for two reasons: first, their interest in dental mercury and second, because of the debilitating nature of environmental illness. In previous chapters, I mentioned that disease may result from a series of reactions in which the body is not able to adapt to its environment; the greater this inability to adapt, the more sick the individual may become. People who have environmental illness react adversely to most substances in their environment, but in a more extreme way. Because of their extreme reaction to most substances, the environmentally ill patient can shed more light on the ill effects of dental mercury than any other group.

The survey sent to environmentally ill patients consisted of two parts. The first part was published in *The Human Ecologist*.[1] This survey asked general dental questions but included specific questions which would provide information on dental amalgam fillings.

The information sought by the first survey included:

1) Whether patients had symptoms of myofacial pain or temporomandibular joint pain,
2) If patients were sensitive to environmental substances,
3) What degenerative diseases patients had,
4) If patients had gum disease,
5) If patients had dental amalgam and/or gold fillings,
6) Whether the patient had any unusual tastes and
7) What the patient's experience was with amalgam replacement.

The second survey was sent to those patients who indicated in the first survey that they had had their dental amalgam fillings replaced. This was done in order to identify their experiences from the replacement procedure. This follow-up survey asked information about:

1) Symptoms that the patient attributed to dental mercury,
2) Tests performed to diagnose mercury allergy or mercury toxicity,
3) Supplements used during and after the amalgam replacement process,
4) Replacement material used,
5) Ill effects during removal of amalgam fillings,
6) Ill effects after replacement of amalgam fillings,
7) What symptoms improved and
8) A chronological list of symptoms and treatment from the beginning of environmental illness until present.

I received 46 responses to the patient survey. Forty-four had been diagnosed as having environmental illness with sensitivities to chemicals, foods, molds, seasonals, dust, mites and Candida. There were a few patients who either didn't know or were not sensitive to mites or dust. Of the 25 patients responding to the question on hypoglycemia, 15 had been diagnosed as having hypoglycemia. Of the 16 patients responding to the question about gum disease, 10 had a history of gum disease. Twelve of the 46 patients indicated that they had both gold and amalgam fillings in their mouths. Fourteen of the 46 patients stated that they were bothered by a metallic taste. However, there was no correlation between having both amalgam and gold fillings and a metallic taste. Twenty-three patients were advised to replace their amalgam fillings and 16 of the 23 complied with that recommendation.

## B. Results of patient surveys

Patients indicated that they had several of the following symptoms before they had their amalgam fillings replaced; they attributed these symptoms to their dental amalgam fillings. The asterisk (*) before the symptom indicates that the symptom was relieved by amalgam replacement.

* a. "Type A" personality (referred to as hyper, driven, perfectionist)
* b. Personality changes
* c. Headache
* d. Confusion
* e. Decreased memory
* f. Lower energy
* g. Fatigue
* h. Weakness
* i. Cravings for foods
* j. Decreased appetite
* k. Indigestion
* l. Metallic taste
* m. Facial pain
* n. Back pain
* o. Seasonal allergies
* p. Petrochemical allergies
* q. Food allergies
  r. Insomnia
* s. Poor stress management
  t. Sensitivity to cold
  u. Bloating

The following symptoms were experienced by some patients during the removal of their amalgam fillings:

a. Brain fag (low mental energy, inability to think)
b. Irritability
c. Dizziness
d. Depression
e. Uncontrollable crying
f. Feeling of impending death
g. Weakness

h. Slow speech
i. Shakiness
j. Rash

The responses by patients who had had their amalgam fillings replaced also varied. The most positive findings were indicated by one multiple sclerosis (MS) patient. She indicated that

> When my fillings were replaced, I no longer needed to take additional supplemental vitamins—especially the B family. I have had *no* MS symptoms as long as I stay away from allergic foods and chemicals. At the end of January, I began T.O.E.[mold immunotherapy] weekly shots for Candida albicans yeast infection. After two of these shots, my vitamin supplements became even less. I have never felt better in 25 years—lots of energy, clear thinking, no facial aches or bad breath. It is unbelievable.

AUTHOR'S NOTE: This patient's history supports the belief that a disease has multiple causes and that the more treatment stones you turn over, the better will be your chances for improvement and the greater the level of health you will achieve.

Another patient indicated that

> I tolerate many more foods and can go out in public more easily. Since I experiment with vitamins, yoga, etc., I can't attribute the improvement directly to the dentistry; though it may have helped significantly, I don't know for sure.

On a less positive note was one patient who wrote that "I would like to say that I am healed after the long ordeal and great expense; but, can only say that I have a little more stamina and a little less sensitivity."

The most recent note that I received from a patient stated that "Just a note to let you know the improvement since I had my amalgams out . . . I can digest my food without difficulty . . . I am still allergic to many things though . . ."

On the negative side, a patient wrote "I experienced a flare-up of my symptoms of the environmental illness from the use of the [Dr. Huggins'] supplements. I cleared rapidly with the cessation of his mineral and vitamin supplements."

The most negative reaction that I received was from a patient who wrote:

> [I had] all my fillings out in one day . . . There was an immediate improvement . . . I could eat foods without feeling

sick . . . I did not realize I would be going into withdrawal as my body tried to throw off the mercury . . . two weeks later . . . I could feel the television's electromagnetic waves . . . The vibrations would make me extremely nervous and I would fall into a drugged sleep. The radio [made me] feel extremely hyper and would get a stiff neck . . . The refrigerator [made me] . . . so nervous I started crying . . . The typewriter [gave me] nose bleeds . . . I craved salt [containing aluminum which] gave me pain in my right arm . . . Taking metal antigen [made] the nervousness stop . . . 10 months later . . . I still have a strong metal sensitivity.

Answers to the other questions in the survey were fairly routine. The tests performed on some patients prior to removal of dental amalgam fillings included blood, urine and hair analyses, mercury patch testing, amalgameter testing and testing of proposed replacement dental materials. However, not all patients had the replacement material tested prior to having those fillings placed.

The supplements used included the "Matrix Minerals" brand of vitamins and minerals and those which can be purchased in health food stores.

The most common replacement filling material was composite followed by gold. Of the many composites available, P30 (3M Company) was the most frequently used. However, several patients did indicate a sensitivity to P30.

## 3. SURVEY OF DENTISTS

### A. Letters and Telephone Calls

I also sent a survey to several dentists who routinely practice mercury-free dentistry in order to obtain feedback from them concerning their methods for the replacement of amalgam fillings. Names of the dentists were obtained from clinical ecologists, Dr. Huggins' office and from Toxic Testing, Inc. Although I did not receive any initial response from the letters that I sent, I did obtain the information contained in this section by telephone interviews with several of the dentists. This information included:

1) Whether the dentists strictly followed Dr. Huggins' protocol for amalgam removal—sequential removal according to amalgameter readings and use of Matrix Minerals Inc. supplements,

2) What filling material was used to replace amalgam fillings,

3) Whether the new filling material was tested for allergic reaction,
4) What brand of supplements were recommended to patients and
5) What other dental procedures and materials were used.

## B. Results of the survey of dentists

Not all of the dentists with whom I spoke strictly adhered to Dr. Huggins' or Mr. Ziff's protocol for the removal of amalgam fillings. The dentists used a variety of methods to determine the sequence for the removal of the amalgam fillings. These methods included: 1) sequential removal determined by amalgameter, 2) removal using the Voll Tooth Chart (acupuncture) and 3) replacement according to the size, number and location of fillings.

The most-used filling materials were the composites P10 or P30 (3M Company) followed by Bio C (Stern) gold. The replacement filling material and the other dental materials were not routinely allergy tested.

Supplementation ranged from the use of Matrix Minerals Inc. vitamins and minerals to supplements purchased by the patient in a health food store. In general, for the patients having acute allergy or acute chemical sensitivity, their physicians managed their supplementation.

Dentists indicated that there was a positive improvement in patients' symptoms resulting from the replacment of amalgam fillings. However, you should be aware that dentists, in general, see very few acutely ill patients for amalgam replacement.

## 4. EVALUATION OF THE SURVEYS

Both clinical ecologists and patients related a wide range of results produced by amalgam replacement. Some clinical ecologists indicated a positive experience with their patients who replaced their amalgam fillings; others indicated negative experiences. Patients, likewise, had a similar range of results. There were success stories following both the anti-mercury protocol and routine amalgam replacement. On the other hand, there were also failures following either method of replacement.

Success occurred most often when the dentist had a full understanding of the patient's medical condition, the physician had a full understanding of dental procedures and dental materials and patients were under strict environmental control so that their only stress was that of dental treatment.

## LOOKING BACK

1. A survey was sent to clinical ecologists, patients and dentists.
2. Clinical ecologists who responded indicated that mercury may contribute to the overall symptomatology of patients with environmental disease, but was only one factor to be considered. The results of the replacement of amalgam fillings were varied with some patients improving and some patients having setbacks. In those patients who improved, there was a 3 to 4-month period during which the frequency of their symptoms increased.
3. The patient survey produced information paralleling that of the clinical ecologists.
4. The responding dentists used varied methods to test for and to replace fillings; some were consistent with the recommendations of the anti-mercury group and some were not. The most frequently used replacement material was composite.

### REFERENCES

1. Fasciana, G.: "EI Dentist Survey," *The Human Ecologist*, #27, p. 13, Fall, 1984.

# 11
# GENERAL
# CONSIDERATIONS

LOOKING AHEAD

1. HEALTH CATEGORIES OF PATIENTS

2. DECIDING ABOUT YOUR DENTAL AMALGAM FILLINGS
   A. Your Health Category
   B. Your Decision About Your Dental Amalgam Fillings
   C. Tests Used To Evaluate Mercury Allergy and Toxicity

3. CHOOSING A REPLACEMENT MATERIAL
   A. Background
   B. General Considerations
   C. Gold as a Replacement Material
   D. Composite as a Replacement Material
   E. Porcelain as a Replacement Material

4. CHOOSING A DENTIST
   A. Background
   B. Whom Do You Go To?

5. REPLACEMENT PROCEDURES
   A. Background
   B. Local Anesthetics
   C. Amalgam Removal
   D. Pulp Medication
   E. Replacement with Composites
   F. Replacement with Gold

LOOKING BACK

## LOOKING AHEAD

After reading the preceding chapters, you are probably pretty close to making a decision about your dental amalgam fillings. If you believe that there is enough evidence to indicate that the mercury in dental amalgam fillings is harmful, you may have already decided that you are going to replace your fillings. On the other hand, if you believe that there is not enough evidence, you might have decided to "wait and see" or to replace your amalgam fillings with mercury-free filling materials as they need to be replaced.

If you are still not sure about your amalgam fillings, this chapter provides you with some additional considerations. Chapter Twelve will provide allergic and environmentally ill patients with specific considerations on the procedures used in amalgam replacement.

## 1. HEALTH CATEGORIES OF PATIENTS

To simplify our discussion, I have divided patients into three categories: healthy, "twixter" and sick. In addition to this arbitrary division, I have listed characteristics which would commonly apply to each category. Although individual patients will not experience all the characteristics of any one group, they will probably experience a good number of them.

Healthy individuals generally do not have any signs or symptoms of disease; they have no complaints and are in good physical and mental condition. Their good physical condition is demonstrated by an adequate amount of energy and a good balance between work and play. Healthy individuals are mentally alert and possess a positive mental attitude. They enjoy a good amount of social interaction, are enthusiastic and enjoy life's challenges. If you were to ask them about their lives, they would indicate that "time flies; I never have enough time to do all the things I'd like to do."

At the other extreme, sick patients have signs and symptoms of disease and have been diagnosed as having one or more recognized diseases. They have complaints, and, depending on the extent of their illnesses, are usually not in as good a physical or mental condition as their healthy counterparts. Their decreased physical condition is demonstrated by an inadequate or inconsistent amount of energy and an excessive interest in rest. Sick individuals are usually preoccupied with their illness; they are less mentally alert than their healthy counterparts. Their negative mental attitude is characteristic of ill health. Individuals who are sick are usually withdrawn and show a general lack of interest. If they are asked about their lives, they may respond that "life is a burden; time drags."

"Twixters" are people who are neither really healthy nor really sick. They generally feel below par. They have fleeting signs and symptoms, but their doctors usually cannot find anything wrong. If the patients persist in their complaints, they may be pronounced "hypochondriac" or their symptoms may be described as "in their head." Twixters fluctuate between periods of having lots of energy and being chronically fatigued; between having enthusiasm and lacking interest; between having a positive mental attitude and having a negative mental attitude. Their socializing interests will vary; in fact, many of the twixters are considered moody. The twixters are characterized as complaining about how they feel, but make excuses as to why they don't feel good. They may say for example, "I don't have any energy at night; I have a lot of tension all day long at work." If you asked them about their lives they probably would say that "I feel like life is passing me by." The plight of the twixters is understandable because they feel good one day and, for no apparent reason, feel poorly the next day.

Identifying your health category is the first step toward making a decision about your dental amalgam fillings and also about other stresses in your life.

## 2. DECIDING ABOUT YOUR DENTAL AMALGAM FILLINGS

### A. Your Health Category

Have you decided what health category most accurately applies to you? Good, your health category decision will help guide you to a decision about your dental amalgam fillings.

Being healthy, you may decide that amalgam replacement is not necessary at this time. If this is your decision, you should always be alert for any danger signals which would notify you that you must reevaluate those things in your life which may be putting a stress on your system and thus jeopardize your health. For instance, if you begin to notice that you have less energy, less enthusiasm or less interest in things, you may want to reevaluate your lifestyle, your nutrition, and your environment. Of course, dental mercury, like other toxins, is part of your environment.

If you are sick, you probably realize by now that disease results from multiple factors and that all stress affects your entire body. Diabetic patients are fooling themselves if then think they are perfectly healthy except for their pancreas. Their entire system is below par. This "below par" just happened to show up first in their pancreas. Knowing this, your desire to regain health should include an evaluation of factors such as your mental attitude, your lifestyle, your nutrition, your genetic weaknesses and your environment. It is a good idea for you to look through the suggested readings in the back of this book to add to your knowledge about the various factors that contribute to disease. Once you have a broad understanding of the disease process, you and your physician can make some decisions which will put you on the right track towards health. Regaining health or maintaining health takes motivation and hard work. It doesn't just happen. Unfortunately, when you are sick, you don't have an awful lot of energy; but, you have to start somewhere. If you want optimum health badly enough, you'll go for it! No achievement feels as good as the sweet victory over illness especially when you know that you took part in the process.

As you have seen, the twixters are the in-between-group. Their mission is easier than that of those individuals who are sick because twixters have more energy and may remember what it feels like to be really healthy. This memory should give you the motivation to make the move towards better health. Don't get discouraged and don't give up until you find the answer to what is making you feel below par. Remember, dental amalgam fillings are only one of the things you should examine if you want to be healthy. If you explore all the possibilities the first time around, you will increase your chances to regain your health. If you don't have time to do right the first time, when will you have time to do it again?

Your children fall into a category by themselves. Because of the literature available about the relationship between dental mercury and health, there is no reason for you to consider putting amalgam fillings in your children's teeth. There are alternative filling materials which are not as controversial as dental amalgam. If I were to decide on a filling material for my children's teeth, I would choose to err on the safe side. If sometime in the future, scientists *prove* that dental amalgam fillings are safe and you had composite fillings put into your children's teeth, you have lost nothing. If the reverse proves to be true, and amalgams are scientifically proven to be unsafe, then you will have made an unnecessary mistake if you put amalgam fillings in your children's teeth.

With children, the best commitment that you can make is to prevent the need for fillings. Knowing what type of diet is good for your teeth will help you to achieve this goal. Interestingly enough, the very diet that is good for you is also good for your teeth. You know what diet I'm talking about—good-bye candy, good-bye sugar, and so forth. Proper oral hygiene is also an essential step in prevention. Among the things that your dentist can do for you and for your children is to apply sealants (plastic coatings) on the chewing surfaces of the back teeth to prevent decay.

### B. *Your Decision About the Mercury in Your Dental Amalgam Fillings*

Your decision to replace your amalgam fillings will also depend on whether you believe that there is enough mercury liberated from your dental fillings to interfere with your body processes and, therefore, interfere with your health. You saw that interference with a single enzyme could produce an autoimmune disease. You saw that toxins in very minute quantities are capable of interfering with certain body processes. You saw that antigens in minute amounts can stimulate your body to react to them. You also saw that toxins are cumulative and that each toxin adds to your total toxic load. This cumulative effect means that toxins in smaller amounts are capable of hurting you.

I also discussed some of the things that you can do to help yourself prevent the effects of toxins, such as diet, exercise, lifestyle and mental attitude.

The bottom line is that you are going to have to make this decision yourself; it is a part of taking charge of your health. In the end, taking charge will make you a better person. If I told you that you *must* replace your amalgam fillings, I would be doing you a disservice. How will you deal with the next health problem that you face? I want you to talk with your physician and your dentist and then make an educated decision. Having to do this might make you feel uncomfortable at first, but you'll get used to it.

### C. *Tests Used to Evaluate Mercury Allergy and Toxicity*

You remember that mercury has two potentially adverse effects: allergic and toxic. If you believe that the mercury liberated from amalgam fillings is toxic, then you don't need to test for mercury allergy. The fact that dental mercury is toxic is enough reason to replace your amalgam fillings. The procedures indicated in the next chapter will offer you the best protection from both a toxic and allergic exposure when you replace your amalgam fillings. In addition, your dentist and physician may want to do blood, urine and hair studies to assess your present health status and to determine if you are excreting mercury once your fillings are removed.

The mercury patch test, used to determine sensitivity to mercury, has little relevance because it is not mercury allergy with which we are most concerned; but *it is the toxicity of mercury which makes dental amalgam an unacceptable dental filling material*. In addition, the mercury patch test itself can sensitize you and/or cause unnecessary exacerbation of symptoms by adding to your toxic load.

Amalgameter testing for sequential removal of amalgam fillings is also unnecessary according to the scientific literature. However, if your dentist believes strongly in sequential removal, I don't see any reason to object to this protocol since it does not cause any harm by itself. I just don't believe it is necessary.

Once you have made the decision to replace your amalgams, the remaining choices are: Who will do the replacement and what replacement material is going to be used? I will discuss the replacement material first.

## 3. CHOOSING A REPLACEMENT MATERIAL

### A. Background

When you decide to replace your amalgam fillings, you will be faced with choosing a replacement dental filling material. Before you and your dentist select a material that is suitable for you, it is helpful for you to understand the process by which dental materials are approved for use in your mouth.

The ADA has two councils (a committee of dentists and allied health professionals) that evaluate dental drugs, materials and equipment: The Council on Dental Therapeutics (CDT) and the Council on Dental Materials, Instruments and Equipment (CDMIE).

The Council on Dental Therapeutics studies and evaluates all drugs and chemicals used in the diagnosis, treatment and prevention of dental disease. These products are given a classification, based on available scientific evidence, of "accepted" (because there is sufficient evidence for safety and effectiveness), "provisionally accepted" (because there is reasonable evidence of usefulness and safety, but lack evidence of dental usefulness) and "unacceptable" (because there is no substantial usefulness or there is a question of safety).

The process by which the CDT evaluates products is as follows:

1) A manufacturer submits a product to the Council for consideration.
2) The Council lists the product as accepted if it meets the standards of acceptance set forth by the Council: usefulness, composition, advertising and labeling.
3) The listing as accepted lasts for three years and is renewable.
4) The product is reviewed whenever new scientific evidence is available.

Second is the Council on Dental Materials, Instruments and Equipment which evaluates dental materials, dental instruments and dental equipment. The CDMIE classifies dental products as "acceptable," "provisionally acceptable" or "certified." A product is classified as acceptable if there is scientific evidence of safety and usefulness established by biological laboratory or clinical evaluation or both. If, in addition to this evaluation, there are physical standards or specifications developed, the product is transferred to the certification program. In this case, the manufacturers certify that their products meet the specifications required by the CDMIE.

What do these classifications mean to you?

If a dental therapeutic agent (drug or chemical) has the classification of "accepted," it means that there is sufficient scientific evidence for its safety and effectiveness. If a dental material is "certified," it means that the product meets the physical standards and specifications required by the ADA. Although this system is a good guide to dental materials and chemicals, it is not foolproof as seen by the "certified" classification given to dental alloys and dental mercury used in amalgam fillings.[1]

AUTHOR'S NOTE: The ADA Councils evaluate dental chemicals and materials according to biological safety. Through personal communications with dental manufacturing companies, I have been told that, for some dental materials and chemicals, the dental manufacturing company concentrates on biocompatibility with the pulp and does not concentrate on biocompatibility with the body.

### B. General Considerations

At the present time, you have three choices for amalgam replacement material: gold, composite and porcelain. Because gold contains different metals and is cemented in place, composites contain many different chemicals and porcelain alternatives have some drawbacks, I have listed some of the more popular filling materials in Appendix IV, Dental Materials. AUTHOR'S NOTE: Porcelain fillings materials have been used as a single filling material and in combination with other materials such as gold and nickel. Because of its lack of strength and brittleness, the use of porcelain by itself has been limited to front teeth (called porcelain jacket crowns) where the compressive forces were low. Some of the new porcelain materials are recommended for posterior (back) teeth. Whether you choose gold, composite or porcelain as a replacement material will depend on the following factors:

   a. The relative allergic potential of the alternative replacement materials.
   b. The relative toxic potential of the alternative replacement materials.
   c. The amount of service you can expect from each filling material.
   d. The cost of each alternative filling material.
   e. The types of other restorative materials already in your mouth.

a. *Relative allergic potential*—All dental materials have allergic potential; some materials have a high allergic potential while others have a low allergic potential. Although gold has the lowest allergic potential, you will have to evaluate the allergic potential of the cements used to hold the gold filling in place. Gold foil, although rarely used, does not need cement to hold it in place. Cast gold fillings, used for inlays, onlays and crowns, contain other metals which should also be evaluated for their allergic potential.

Composites consist of chemical compounds (called a monomer) which are capable of "holding hands" with each other to form a larger molecule (called a polymer). Composites also contain fillers (e.g., quartz and glass) and other chemical compounds which control specific characteristics of the material. These characteristics enable composite material to be used as a dental filling material. Composites give off chemicals while they are setting (getting hard); they are also subject to wear. During this wear, composites give off minute chemical compounds.

Porcelain consists of feldspar (potassium aluminum silicate), silica (quartz or flint) and kaolin (clay). To allow your dentist to match the shade of the filling to your own tooth, coloring pigments are added to the porcelain powder. These pigments include titanium oxide, manganese oxide, iron oxide, cobalt oxide, copper oxide, chromium oxide or nickel oxide. Tin oxides are used to increase opacity. Porcelain restorations are considered to be stable; none of the ingredients are believed to leak out of the filling. Because of its stability, porcelain is not thought to contribute to allergies. Of course the cements used to hold the porcelain filling should be evaluated.

Allergies to composites have been reported in scientific literature; because of this, an allergy evaluation of composites should be done if you have a high tendency towards allergy. You should be aware that if you do not have an adverse reaction to the allergy testing of a dental material this does not mean that you won't develop an allergy to it at some time in the future. If your body is working properly, allergy to filling materials is less likely.

b. *Relative toxic potential*—All dental materials are chemicals and, as such, have some toxic potential. Gold has the lowest toxic potential. However, gold filling materials (inlays, onlays and crowns) contain other metals which have to be evaluated because of their toxic potential. This is discussed later in this chapter in the section "Gold as a Replacement Material."

As you read in the last section, composites give off compounds as they wear. These organic compounds can be chemically changed in your body. This change makes it difficult to follow these compounds as they travel throughout your body. Because the new compounds are difficult to identify, it is unknown if composites are toxic. Any dental material can be toxic depending on the individual. What you must consider is the relative toxicity. A review of the literature indicates that mercury is a known toxin; the literature has not addressed the toxic potential of composites.

If porcelain has any toxic potential, it is due to the minute quantities of pigments that are added. The pigments that have toxic potential are cobalt and nickel.

c. *Amount of service you can expect*—The use that a dental filling provides is called its service. This service depends on three interrelated factors: the type of filling material, the quality of the filling material and the suitability (professional judgment) of the filling material to the patient's medical/dental condition. There are some general guidelines involved in selecting a filling material. If there is little decay and the filling needed is small, a filling material of lesser strength can be chosen. As the amount of decay gets larger, and, because of this, the remaining tooth structure gets smaller, a stronger filling material is needed. In the first case, the tooth is strong enough to hold the filling in place; in the second case, a filling material is needed to provide strength for the tooth. In the past, amalgam would have been selected for the former and gold for the latter. With amalgam out of the picture, composite is chosen for the former and gold is chosen for the latter.

An additional factor to consider is the relative wear capacity of the filling material. Because of its hardness, gold gives superior wear. On the other hand, composites, being softer than gold, wear more poorly.

Another important quality of a filling material is called marginal integrity. This simply means that the margin of the filling (where the filling meets the tooth) should remain intact in order to prevent recurrent decay, sensitivity and pupal damage. Gold is excellent in this area; however, with the new bonding techniques, composites also have excellent marginal integrity.

Each type of filling material comes in a variety of qualities. In general, companies with the best reputations produce superior products.

Your dentist considers each of these factors prior to recommending a suitable filling material for you. His professional judgment takes into account your medical health (whether you have allergies, diabetes or any other condition), your general dental health (whether you have gum disease, abscesses or some other dental disease), your bite (how your teeth mesh together), whether you have any missing teeth (if you need a partial denture or bridgework to restore your chewing), how large a filling is needed and what your desires are for your dental health. When all these factors are put together, you can expect the greatest service from the dollars which you spend on your dental treatment.

d. *Cost*—Gold is the most expensive filling material used by your dentist, but it is also the longest-lasting. If you have gold inlays, onlays or crowns done, *and* you take care of your teeth, you can expect to have excellent service from your dental care. Porcelain fillings cost about what gold fillings cost since porcelain fillings involve the same steps as gold fillings. The cost of dental treatment is an important factor because gold fillings can cost as much as three to four times that of composite fillings.

e. *Types of other filling materials present in your mouth*—Another factor which you must evaluate is the presence of different metals in your mouth (gold, amalgam and metallic partial dentures). Even if you decide not to replace your amalgam fillings, there is evidence that having both gold and amalgam in your mouth at the same time can increase the potential for health problems. The reason for this is the difference in the electrical potential between the different metals. This difference in electrical potential is said to increase the amount of mercury liberated from the amalgam fillings. Because metallic partial dentures contain several metals, they must be evaluated as well. When possible, it is prudent to have the least number of metals in your mouth at the same time. It may be a good idea to have partial dentures made of gold if you have gold fillings already in place. There is no information in the literature to indicate that you should not have both composite and gold in your mouth at the same time.

A final note of caution: a few years ago, during the "gold crisis," non-precious crowns (caps) were being recommended due to the high cost of gold. These non-precious materials contained nickel which has since been identified as an allergen and as a toxin. For this reason, it is wise to replace that type of restorative material.

## C. Gold as a Replacement Material

Before amalgam was introduced to dentistry, gold was used almost exclusively. Gold has been used for about 2500 years, first in a crude fashion to replace teeth which had been extracted (pulled) and later in a more refined way as a filling material. Replacement of missing teeth was a joint effort by physicians, barber-surgeons, goldsmiths and artisans. Individual fillings were fabricated from gold leaf (similar to gold foil).

Because gold is a soft metal, it is combined with other metals to produce characteristics which are suitable for different applications in dentistry. For instance, a small cavity which is not on the chewing surface of a tooth can be filled with a "soft" gold alloy. (An alloy is a combination of two or more metals.) On the other hand, a crown (cap) which is designed to strengthen the tooth needs a "harder" gold.

When used in dentistry, gold is combined with one or more of the following metals: silver, copper, platinum, palladium and zinc, but can contain other metals as well. Gold is considered a noble metal, but, as an alloy, it becomes less noble as it is combined with non-noble metals. Noble means that the metal is resistant to oxidation, tarnish and corrosion. Other noble metals used in dentistry are palladium and platinum. These noble metals, together with silver, are called precious metals. There is a distinction between noble and precious. Because silver corrodes, it is considered a precious metal, but not a noble metal; palladium and platinum are considered both noble and precious.

1) *The use of other metals*—Other metals are added to gold in order to alter its characteristics so that it can be used in a wider variety of applications. Platinum, for example, adds to the hardness and elastic qualities of the gold. Silver neutralizes the reddish color of yellow gold alloys containing appreciable quantities of copper. Copper gives the alloy strength and hardness.

2) *"Types" of gold*—A discussion of the "types" of gold will help you to further understand the combination of other metals with

gold. There are four types of gold: Type I, Type II, Type III and Type IV. Each type of gold has a specific purpose for its use in inlays, onlays, crowns, bridge abutments (the tooth that holds the bridge) and removable partial dentures. The types of gold and their use is outlined below:

| Type | Hardness | Filling Design |
|------|----------|----------------|
| I | soft | dental inlays |
| II | medium | inlays needing more strength |
| III | hard | onlays and single crowns |
| IV | extra hard | fixed bridgework |
| | | or removable partial dentures |

3) *Choice of gold*—The filling design determines what "type" of gold is used. For small fillings on the sides of the teeth, it is acceptable to use Type I gold. For long bridges, it is necessary to use Type IV gold. Many companies offer these different types of gold. However, because different gold products contain a variety of metals, we'll have to pay attention to the contents as well as the type of gold. Ideally, the more noble the metal, the less corrosion we can expect. The fewer the metals, the less electrical complications will occur. As you can see, asking for gold fillings is not specific enough. We must be concerned with what other metals are used and what their health implications are.

### D. Composite as a Replacement Material

Composites are the "white" filling materials usually used in the front teeth. They can contain either the compound bis-phenol glycidyl methacrylate (BIS-GMA) and/or urethane dimethacrylate as the monomer. When one molecule of these compounds is made to chemically react with other like molecules, the material forms a large molecule (polymer) composed of these units of BIS-GMA or urethane dimethacrylate. These units are chemically joined and cannot be separated under ordinary circumstances. The molecules are made to react with each other either by mixing an activator (e.g., benzoyl peroxide) with the material or by having a light sensitive activator in the material (e.g., benzoin ethyl ether). In the latter case, a special light (white or ultraviolet) is placed next to the filling material, the filling material is hardened by undergoing a chemical reaction called polymerization.

Composite filling materials contain fillers which give them strength, color and water resistance. These fillers can include quartz, borosilicate glass, lithium aluminum silicate, barium aluminum silicate and barium fluoride. The composite Trans-Lit (Merz + Co.) is a product made from oyster shells; it contains "0.02% mercury amidochloride."

Until recently, composites were considered suitable only in filling situations where there was no pressure on the filling. Improvements in the materials and the techniques of applying those materials to the tooth have made composites suitable for some posterior (back teeth used for chewing) teeth. Although they are not the best choice, composites can replace amalgam fillings in a great many situations.

Composites have a shorter life expectancy than gold because they are subject to wear and breakage.

Since composite material is not as strong as gold or amalgam, is subject to shrinkage, and does not possess a high marginal integrity, the method of application of the filling material is important to minimize these shortcomings. For these reasons, bonding has become very popular in recent years. Bonding simply means that the filling material is made to "bond" with the tooth. Bonding is accomplished by a technique called acid-etching. Acid-etching involves applying a suitable weak acid, usually phosphoric, to the enamel of the tooth. After 30–60 seconds, the solution is washed off. This etching removes some of the minerals in the enamel and gives the enamel a dull (matte) finish. A thin coat of unbilled composite material is painted over the cavity preparation. This layer bonds to the tooth enamel and to the filling. This process improves the marginal integrity, reduces the possibility of recurrent decay along the margin, and increases retention.

Composites have the ability to bond the tooth together in order to strengthen the integrity of the tooth to resist cusp breakage.

### E. Porcelain as a Replacement Material

The use of porcelain for crowning posterior teeth is relatively new. Porcelain is thought to be biocompatible. Although porcelain is not as strong as gold, it is considerably stronger than composites. The shortcoming of porcelain is its brittleness—it may be broken or cracked.

## 4. CHOOSING A DENTIST

### A. Background

I decided to discuss choosing a dentist after choosing a replacement dental material because your choice of a dentist may depend on your dental needs. For example, if you have very large fillings, possibly one or more missing teeth and have a history of myofacial pain (pain in the temple or chewing muscles) or temporomandibular joint dysfunction (pain, clicking and pathology in the temporomandibular joint—just inside the front of your ear), you may want to go to a prosthodontist. A prosthodontist is a dentist who specializes in replacing missing teeth with bridgework, or badly broken down teeth with crowns (caps), inlays or onlays. He also has additional training in occlusion (the way that your teeth come together when you chew).

### B. Whom do you go to?

There are two important criteria in choosing a dentist: first, the dentist does good dental work and second, there is open communication between you and your dentist. You may already have a family dentist with both of these qualities. If you do, you need not look any further. Your dentist does not have to agree with the position that amalgam fillings pose a health hazard, but he or she must be open-minded and willing to take the steps necessary to satisfactorily replace your amalgam fillings.

If you don't have a dentist, how do you go about choosing one? I wrote a fairly comprehensive article on "Choosing a Dentist" for *The Human Ecologist*. This article is reproduced in the booklet entitled *Dental Materials: An Outline for the Allergic and Chemically Sensitive Patients*; I will summarize it here.

Once you know what level of dental health you want, a good starting place to secure a dentist is with your family physician. In addition to your physician, you may ask friends, relatives, co-workers or other people who have had similar dental treatment accomplished. Perhaps your eye doctor, your pharmacist or your child's pediatrician may be able to help. Once you get a couple of names, you should make an appointment to speak with the dentist to determine how cooperative you may expect him or her to be. It may be a good idea to go in person to the office to make this appointment. If the individuals who recommended the dentist are reliable and your impression of the dentist and his staff are favorable, you may be on your way. If during your consultation with the dentist, you feel that you are not going to get the cooperation that you need, keep looking. Remember, a good operator *and* cooperation are both important.

# 5. REPLACEMENT PROCEDURES

## A. Background

The procedures used by your dentist depend on what replacement material is suitable for you. The procedures used for gold fillings are the same as for porcelain fillings. The procedures used for both gold and porcelain are completely different from procedures used for composite fillings with the exception of anesthetic agents and amalgam removal. I will present each procedure after a general discussion of local anesthetics and amalgam removal.

## B. Local Anesthetics

Anesthetics are chemical agents that prevent sensation by blocking the action of specific nerves. This blocking results in the feeling of numbness. When this blockage is confined to a small, specific area, it is called local anesthesia.

The anesthetic solutions which your dentist uses generally contain three ingredients: an anesthetic agent, a vasoconstrictor and preservatives. The anesthetic agent is the active ingredient which blocks the action of the nerve. Examples of this type of anesthetic solution are Procaine, Lidocaine and Mepivacaine. A vasoconstrictor is sometimes added to the anesthetic solution to reduce the blood flow to the anesthetized nerve. This reduced blood flow allows the anesthetic agent to remain in contact with the nerve for a longer period of time, thereby prolonging the period of anesthesia. Examples of vasoconstrictors are epinephrine, norepinephrine and levonordefrin. Preservatives are present in almost all local anesthetics and can cause hypersensitivity reactions. Please note that the chart below lists preservatives. However the container should be inspected to determine the preservative contained in the anesthetic solution. Some brand names may change preservatives and some generic brands do not contain the same preservatives as the brand name anesthetic (see Table 3).

Your dentist can choose from a wide variety of anesthetic solutions. There are many local anesthetic agents for use by physicians and dentists; in deciding which anesthetic solution to use, your dentist takes into account 1) how long it takes to produce numbness (onset), 2) how long the numbness will last (duration), 3) how toxic the anesthetic is and 4) what adverse reactions the anesthetic may cause. Since dentists need an anesthetic which is fast acting and lasts between 30 to 120 minutes, their choices are limited.

**Table 3: ANESTHETICS**

| Brand | Vasoconstrictor | Preservative | Type | Duration |
|---|---|---|---|---|
| Alphacaine 2% | None | None | Amide | Medium |
| Alphacaine 2% | Epinephrine | Sodium metabisulfite | Amide | Long |
| Lidocaine 2% | None | None | Amide | Medium |
| Lidocaine 2% | Epinephrine | Sodium metabisulfite | Amide | Long |
| Octocaine 2% | Epinephrine | Sodium bisulfite | Amide | Long |
| Xylocaine 2% | Epinephrine | Sodium metabisulfite | Amide | Long |
| Arestocaine 3% | None | None | Amide | Short |
| Arestocaine 2% | Levonordefrin | Acetone sodium bisulfite | Amide | Long |
| Carbocaine 3% | None | None | Amide | Short |
| Carbocaine 2% | Neo-Cobefrin | Acetone sodium bisulfite | Amide | Long |
| Isocaine 3% | None | None | Amide | Short |
| Isocaine 2% | Levonordefrin | Sodium bisulfite | Amide | Long |
| Mepivacaine 3% | None | None | Amide | Short |
| Mepivacaine 2% | Levonordefrin | Sodium metabisulfite | Amide | Long |
| Marcaine 0.5% | Epinephrine | Sodium bisulfite | Amide | Long |
| Citaneste Forte | Epinephrine | Sodium metabisulfite | Amide | Medium |
| Citanest Plain | None | None | Amide | Short |
| Ravocaine | Levophed | Acetone sodium bisulfite | Ester | Long |
| Ravocaine | Neo-Cobefred | Acetone sodium bisulfite | Ester | Long |
| Novocaine | Levophed | Acetone sodium bisulfite | Ester | Medium |
| Novocaine | Neo-Cobefrin | Acetone sodium bisulfite | Ester | Medium |

Anesthetics are categorized by their chemical type (ester or amide), where they are broken down in the body (liver or plasma) and how long they last. The type of anesthetic which is used is important for allergy patients; if you are allergic to one of the "amide" anesthetics, you should only use one of the "ester" types and vice-versa. The part of the body which breaks down the anesthetic agent is important because the anesthetic's toxicity may cause a problem with people who are sick (e.g., liver disease). If a patient has liver disease, an "ester" type of anesthetic may be a good choice for anesthetic agent because ester types of anesthetics are broken down in the plasma. Finally, the length of time that the anesthetic agent produces numbness can be extended by the use of vasoconstrictors. The most popular type of anesthetic agents are listed in Table 3.

Both acupuncture anesthesia (needles placed in critical areas of the body to produce the loss of sensation in another part of the body) and hypnosis (artificially produced trance-like state of sleep) have both been successfully used in dentistry. However, local injection of anesthetic agents is the usual course of treatment.

The choice of anesthetic agent will also depend on the patient's medical condition (e.g., allergy, liver disease) and the length of time needed to complete the dental procedure.

### C. Amalgam Removal

Once your teeth are anesthetized, the old amalgam fillings are removed. During amalgam removal the drilling processes produce mercury vapor as well as fine-ground amalgam particles. In order to minimize your exposure to mercury, researchers recommend the use of a "rubber dam" and "high-speed suction."

A rubber dam is a very thin square piece of rubber (4½ inches). The dentist punches holes into the rubber dam to allow your teeth to go through. This rubber dam is then placed in your mouth. Each tooth in the quadrant receiving treatment is put through the hole prepared for it. This technique isolates the teeth and prevents you from swallowing any amalgam.

A high-speed suction, which resembles a large straw is placed near the tooth which is being drilled. The dental drill gives off a stream of water which washes the debris from the tooth. The debris and water are immediately removed with the high-speed suction.

Once the amalgam fillings are removed and the teeth are medicated, the rubber dam can be taken off if gold fillings are to be done or left in place if composite fillings are to be done.

## D. Pulp Medication

The pulp of the tooth is that part of the tooth which contains the nerves and blood vessels. It extends from the center of the crown of the tooth narrowing to the tip of the root.

PARTS OF THE TOOTH:

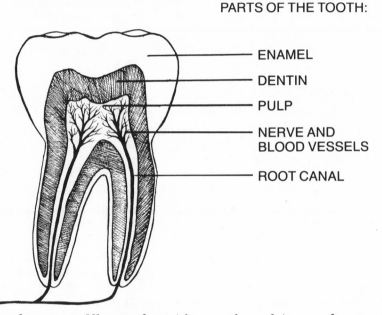

ENAMEL

DENTIN

PULP

NERVE AND BLOOD VESSELS

ROOT CANAL

If the decay or a filling is deep (close to the pulp), a medication is placed in the filling preparation before the filling is inserted. This medication is usually composed of calcium hydroxide. The purpose of calcium hydroxide is to stimulate the pulp to repair the damage caused by the decay or tooth preparation and also for protection and insulation.

## E. Replacement With Composite

Once the amalgam has been removed and the tooth is medicated, the tooth is prepared for the filling. Placing the composite filling involves five main steps: 1) etching the enamel, 2) placing the bonding material on the enamel, 3) placing the filling material into the preparation, 4) initiating the hardening of the filling material and 5) contouring the filling.

1) *Etching*—Once the pulp is protected, the etching gel usually phosphoric acid, is placed on the enamel. After 30 to 60 seconds, the gel is rinsed. This leaves a matte finish (due to the demineralization of

the enamel surface) and prepares the tooth for the bonding material (unfilled composite).

2) *Bonding*—The bonding material is placed on the enamel and dentin and allowed to harden (self-hardening material is called auto-cure material). If a light-cured bonding material is used, it is hardened by shining a special light (white or ultraviolet) on the material.

3) *Placement of the filling*—The filling material is then placed into the cavity preparation.

4) *Hardening*—Once the filling material has been placed in the cavity preparation, it is shaped, contoured and then hardened by use of a special light. The light is held next to the filling material for about 30 to 60 seconds depending on the material (auto-cure filling material is mixed and put into the preparation and then held in place until it hardens).

5) *Contouring*—The filling is then contoured (shaped) to replace the tooth structure which was lost through decay or through the removal of the old filling. The bite is checked to be sure that the filling is properly adjusted.

This entire process for one tooth takes between 30 and 60 minutes depending on the location of the tooth, size of the filling and the difficulty in placing and contouring the filling.

### F. Replacement With Gold

Once the amalgam filling has been removed and the tooth is medicated, the gold filling preparation is done. Because the gold filling is going to be inserted into the preparation in a solid piece, the preparation must be very precise and specially designed with slightly divergent walls.

Placing the gold filling involves more steps than that of the composite filling. The steps involved in placing a gold filling include: 1) taking an impression of the prepared tooth and the opposing teeth (e.g., lower teeth if an upper tooth is being prepared), 2) making a temporary filling (usually acrylic), 3) temporarily cementing the temporary filling, 4) fitting the gold filling and 5) permanently cementing the gold filling. The process takes two two- to three-hour visits.

1) *Taking an impression*—Once the tooth has been prepared for the gold filling, an impression is taken of the tooth. This impression

is used to make a model of the tooth on which the dental laboratory technician can fabricate the gold filling.

2) *The temporary filling*—Because it takes the dental laboratory several days to complete the gold filling, a temporary filling is made of acrylic material to replace the tooth structure lost through decay or through the removal of the old filling.

3) *Temporary cementation of the temporary filling*—The temporary filling (also an inlay) is cemented in place with temporary cement; this cement is softer than permanent cement in order to allow the temporary filling to be easily removed.

4) *Fitting the gold filling*—The gold filling is placed in the prepared tooth. The margins are then fitted to the tooth so that they are smooth. The bite is checked and adjusted if necessary.

5) *Permanent cementation*—The gold filling is then cemented in place and the bite is checked again. The margins are "burnished" (rubbed) so that the margins are perfectly flush against the enamel of the tooth.

## LOOKING BACK

1. People fall into one of three health categories: healthy, sick and "twixters."
2. Your decision on whether to replace your amalgam fillings depends, in part, on which category you believe you fall into.
3. Various tests for mercury toxicity and mercury allergy may not be necessary to formulate your opinion about your amalgam fillings.
4. Choosing a replacement material depends on the relative allergic potential, toxic potential, length of service and cost of the replacement materials. Other types of metal fillings or partial dentures you may have will also influence this choice.
5. In choosing a dentist, ability and cooperation are important.

### REFERENCES

1. Compiled from the Journal of the American Dental Association, (JADA, 109:821, November, 1984), *Accepted Dental Therapeutics*, (American Dental Association, Chicago, 1984) and personal correspondence with dental manufacturing companies.
2. "Clinical Products in Dentistry," *JADA*, 109:821–864, November 1984.

# 12
# SPECIAL
# CONSIDERATIONS

LOOKING AHEAD

1. SHOULD YOU REPLACE YOUR AMALGAM FILLINGS?

2. DENTAL PROCEDURES AND MATERIALS

3. ADDITIONAL FACTORS TO CONSIDER

LOOKING BACK

## LOOKING AHEAD

When you think about going to the dentist, the first thought that comes into your mind is "I hope my dentist doesn't hurt." Until this time, the average dental patient was primarily concerned with whether his or her dentist was going to hurt him/her (cause pain). Today, despite many advances, the average patient is still concerned about pain. However, the "hurt" has taken on a new meaning. This "hurt" now includes adverse medical reactions.

Allergic and environmentally ill patients (EI patients) have had to be concerned with whether their environment was hurting them. They must now be concerned with whether their dental treatment is hurting them. Unlike most patients, allergic and EI patients can be hurt by more substances in the dental office because of their acute sensitivity. Although I have discussed some of these substances in this book, I want to discuss further some dental procedures and dental materials in this chapter. *A WORD OF CAUTION: Allergic and EI patients react differently to the substances in their environment and must consult with their physician prior to beginning any treatment.* Sometimes we may have to compromise on strict avoidance of substances if the long-term value of their use outweighs the adverse effects of a short-term exposure.

## 1. SHOULD YOU REPLACE YOUR AMALGAM FILLINGS?

As you have seen before, both allergic and environmentally ill patients have maladapted responses to their environment. The difference between them is a question of degree of maladaption. What applies to the environmentally ill applies to allergic individuals as well. Someone with only slight allergies may not have to be as careful with dental procedures and dental materials since they are probably more healthy than EI patients.

Dr. Alan Levin describes environmental illness as "Immune System Dysregulation." In other words, environmental illness is the result of an immune system gone awry. Drs. Randolph, Truss, Philpott, Saifer, Crook, Zamm and others indicate that toxins from various sources (chemicals, infection and pollution) can adversely affect your immune system (see Recommended Readings). My research indicates that dental mercury should be put on this list of toxins which cause adverse reactions on the immune system.

If you have several allergies, you should consider replacing your amalgam fillings since there is evidence that the mercury in dental amalgam affects the immune system. If you have environmental illness, it is not a question of "IF" you should replace your amalgam fillings, but "WHEN," "HOW," "WITH WHAT" and "BY WHOM" your fillings are to be replaced.

### 1) *When* Should Your Amalgam Fillings Be Replaced?

The time to replace your amalgam fillings will depend on both your dental history and your general health. If your recent dental history reflects a direct relationship between having a dental amalgam filling placed and some adverse reaction, you may want to remove the offending amalgam filling as soon as possible. If your past dental history reflects a correlation between the placement of dental amalgam fillings and the beginning of some symptoms, you may want to replace all of your amalgam fillings as soon as possible. If you have had a gold filling placed in your mouth along with amalgam fillings and you have experienced symptoms some time after that, you may want to replace your amalgam fillings. If you have had a history of reactions to any mercury-containing compound (merthiolate, mercurochrome and others), you may want to replace your amalgam fillings in the near future. You can see that the speed with which you may want to replace your amalgam fillings depends, in part, on your dental history. Remember, take your time; you may have been sick a long time, another couple of weeks or months isn't going to matter. If you go too fast, you may have a bigger setback than you expect.

How soon you are able to replace your amalgam fillings depends on your general health. Because dental treatment is a traumatic experience and will probably cause some symptoms, you should be in as stable a medical condition as possible before attempting to have your fillings replaced. How do you know if you are in a stable condition? A good indication of stability is being able to go about your daily routine while remaining symptom-free. Another indicator is the time you take to bounce back after an exposure to chemicals, molds or other allergens. For example, if it takes you four to five days to bounce back after a brief exposure to perfume, it will be very difficult for you to sit in a dental office for three to four hours. If you are still testing foods or seasonals, you may want to wait until you are stabilized with your diet and your immunotherapy. You may also want to evaluate and treat any metabolic deficiencies prior to beginning treatment. Depending on how "strong" you are, you should have the following factors under control before you begin amalgam replacement:

a. You should be able to avoid all chemicals which cause symptoms.

b. You should be able to avoid all inhalants (pollen, mold, perfume) which cause symptoms.
c. You should have your immunotherapy program under control.
d. You should have your nutritional program under control (rotary diet, digestive aids, metabolic support and supplements).
e. You should have any infections under control (Candida).
f. You should have your home situation under control—no chemicals, no mold.
g. You should be strong enough to undertake the dental procedures without getting sick.
h. You should have any other medical condition under control (e.g., diabetes).

In general, *you should have only to deal with the stress of dental treatment at the time of amalgam replacement*. When you are able to go through a normal week without symptoms, you are ready to consider amalgam replacement. Remember, the first appointment on Monday morning is best because the dental office has had time to "gas out."

2) *HOW* SHOULD YOU REPLACE YOUR AMALGAM FILLINGS?

A rubber dam must be used when you have your amalgam fillings removed. The use of the rubber dam minimizes your exposure to mercury vapor and amalgam particles. If you are going to replace your fillings with gold, you should have the entire left or right side (top and bottom) done at the same time. This routine should then be followed on the other side. A good plan would be to prepare all the fillings on the left side (or right side) followed by the insertion of those fillings three to four weeks later. On the day following the insertion of these gold fillings, the right side (or left side) should be prepared for gold fillings. This procedure prevents your gold fillings from touching your amalgam fillings and also minimizes the amount of time (one day) in which you would have both gold and amalgam in your mouth. The total procedure for gold fillings may involve four five- to six-hour appointments.

If you are going to replace your amalgam fillings with composites, you may decide to do a quadrant at a time (e.g., upper left). Always give yourself adequate time to bounce back. This "rest" time will minimize your reactions to the dental procedures and dental materials and will thereby minimize your symptoms.

### 3) WITH WHAT SHOULD YOU REPLACE YOUR AMALGAM FILLINGS?

The material having the lowest toxic potential and the lowest allergic potential is gold. A close second is porcelain. It is important to evaluate the cements that are used to hold your gold or porcelain fillings in place. Gold is considered to be the superior filling material.

However, not all dental gold is the same. Because there are different metals added to dental gold to enhance specific characteristics (e.g., hardness), these added metals will have to be evaluated. An important caution about fabricating gold fillings is that the laboratory should be instructed not to mix other gold products with the gold product that you and your dentist have specified for your fillings.

Composite dental filling material is a suitable replacement material in a good number of circumstances. Composites can be used along with gold fillings in the same patient. Many allergists believe that you should evaluate composite filling materials for their allergic potential.

### 4) BY WHOM SHOULD YOUR AMALGAM FILLINGS BE REPLACED?

As I have discussed in other sections, both the ability and the cooperation of your dentist are important. The importance of your dentist's ability speaks for itself. Your dentist's cooperation is important if you are going to minimize your symptoms during and after the dental procedures.

## 2. DENTAL PROCEDURES AND MATERIALS

I will discuss the important procedures and materials you are likely to encounter in a typical dental visit in which a filling will be replaced.

1) *Anesthesia*—As I indicated in the last chapter, there are two classes of anesthetic agents: the ester type and the amide type. The ester type is broken down in the plasma, and the amide type is broken down in the liver. All anesthetics are toxins. However, proceeding with dental treatment without using anesthesia may produce some undesired physiological effects (e.g., stress, changes in body chemistry) which may also temporarily hurt you. The dentist's goal in anesthesia should be to minimize the toxic effect of the anesthetic agent on their patients. They can accomplish this goal in several ways: first, the patient should be assessed in order to determine which class of anesthetic agent will be more suitable to use;

second, the minimal amount of anesthesia should be used to provide the desired numbness; third, adequate time should be allowed for the patient to detoxify the anesthetic agent; and fourth, the patient's exposure to other toxins during the dental procedures should be minimized.

I want to further clarify the third factor. The use of a vasoconstrictor (e.g., epinephrine) in the anesthetic solution will reduce blood flow to the area of injection. This reduced blood flow allows the anesthetic to remain in contact with the nerve over a longer time. Because the anesthetic agent is held in the area of injection over a longer period of time, the amount of anesthetic your body has to detoxify at any one time is lower. For example, if you are given 2 cc of an anesthetic solution which lasts for 20 minutes, your body will take approximately 30 minutes to detoxify the solution. If a vasoconstrictor, which holds the anesthetic solution in the area of injection for 90 minutes, is added then that same amount of anesthetic agent will be detoxified in approximately 100 to 120 minutes.

A disadvantage of using a vasoconstrictor is that the vasoconstrictor itself may be toxic and/or may produce side effects. Epinephrine, for example, may cause nervousness, rapid pulse and rapid heart beat especially in allergic and environmentally ill patients.

Preservatives are sometimes used in anesthetic solutions. These have been known to cause adverse reactions. Among the worst offenders are bisulfite preservatives. The FDA has recently banned the use of bisulfites in foods, but this does not apply to anesthetic solutions.

Which anesthetic solution you and your dentist choose and whether you use a vasoconstrictor should be evaluated by your physician.

Dr. Alfred Zamm, Kingston, New York, recommends *Carbocaine Plain* (Cook and Waite Co.) in individual carpules.[1] Carbocaine comes with and without the vasoconstrictor levonordefrin (1-aminoethyl,3,4 dihydroxybenzyl alcohol).

2) *Amalgam Removal*—Amalgam removal must always take place using the *rubber dam* in order to minimize your exposure to mercury. Breathing in the fumes of the rubber dam may be a temporary inconvenience. Dr. Zamm also suggests breathing with a *nasal mask* containing an oxygen flow to two liters per minute.[1]

3) *High-Speed Suction*—The high-speed suction should always be used during the removal of amalgam fillings and at all times when solvents or other chemicals are used in the mouth. The use of the high-speed suction allows the dentist to evacuate (remove) amalgam

particles and all chemicals from your mouth, thereby minimizing your exposure to these materials.

4) *Drying Agents*—Drying agents are chemicals used to degrease, clean and dry the tooth preparation before the filling is placed. Three popular brands of drying agents used by dentists are: CaviDry (Parkell) which contains methyl ethyl ketone and ethyl acetate, Cavilax (Premier) which contains ethyl acetate and 2-butanone, and Prep-dry (Lee Pharmaceutical) which contains acetone. These agents may be used to clean and dry the preparation before placing a filling. This is especially useful prior to cementing gold fillings. These agents can also produce some inflammation of the pulp; they should be used sparingly and used while the high-speed suction is in working. Drying agents are potentially allergenic agents.

5) *Impression Materials*—Impression materials are used to make models of your teeth when gold fillings are chosen to replace amalgam fillings. There are various types of impression materials. The alginate type of impression material (sodium alginate, flavorings and colorings) is used for an initial impression. Although the quickest, alginate doesn't have the dimensional stability of other impression materials. A relative of alginate impression material is alginate hydrocolloid. This material is extremely accurate and is considered to be a very good impression material for gold fillings. Both alginate and alginate hydrocolloid are fairly safe impression materials for the allergic and EI patient.

The other three types of impression materials include: polysulfide rubber (polysulfide polymer, mercaptan, dibutyl phthalate, oils and stearic acid); silicone rubber (poly-dimethylsiloxane, orthoalkyl-silicate, organic ester, tin octoate or dibutyl tin dilaurate) and polyether rubber (polyether and sulfonic acid). Which one your dentist may use will depend on experience and knowledge as to which material provides the best results. These three products contain volatile chemicals and solvents which may cause you to react adversely. In addition, the time they take to set up in your mouth is about 7 to 9 minutes. Because the success of a gold filling depends, in part, on an accurate impression of the tooth, you may have to compromise on your attempt to avoid these materials if your dentist believes that he can work best with one of them. Note: sulfonates contained in polyether impression materials are extremely allergenic.

6) *Temporary Filling Materials*—Temporary filling materials are used to fill the tooth while the gold filling is being fabricated. Temporary filling materials belong in the category of plastic filling

materials. Temporary filling materials are chemically similar to denture base materials, but their hardening is accelerated by chemicals. Temporary filling materials contain methylmethacrylate, benzoyl peroxide, butyl phthalate, hydroquinone, ethyl glycol dimethacrylate and sometimes methyl p-toluidine.

When temporary filling materials are used, they should be prepared in a room other than the room you are in. Preferably, the material (liquid and powder) should be mixed completely outside the dental office. The mixed material should *never* be placed in your mouth until it is hardened and until all of the liquid has either evaporated or reacted with the powder. The temporary filling should be made on a model, not in your mouth. This is one step in which you can avoid a very large chemical exposure.

7) *Temporary Cements*—Temporary cements are used to hold the temporary filling in place for a short period of time (1 to 2 weeks) while the gold filling is being fabricated. These cements must be strong enough to hold the temporary filling in place but weak enough to allow the easy removal of the temporary filling when necessary. Temporary cements come in two types: those containing eugenol and those which do not contain eugenol. Because eugenol is an oil extracted from cloves and adversely affects some patients, the eugenol-free temporary cements should be considered. Nogenol (Coe Company) is eugenol-free but does contain peppermint oil and peanut oil.

8) *Permanent Cements*—The finished gold filling is cemented into place using a permanent cement. The four general categories of permanent cements are: zinc phosphate cement (zinc oxide and orthophosphoric acid); EBA cement (zinc oxide, eugenol and ethyoxybenzoic acid); polycarboxylate cements (zinc oxide, aluminum oxide, stannous fluoride and polyacrylic acid) and acrylic resin cements (methylmethacrylate and benzoyl peroxide). Of these cements, zinc phosphate cement is preferred because it is composed of inorganic materials which are less likely to produce adverse reactions. The pulp must be protected prior to using zinc phosphate and silicophosphate cements since they are acids.

9) *Pulp Protection*—The pulp needs to be protected from the chemicals used in dental procedures and from some of the dental materials themselves. There are two agents used for pulp protection: cavity varnish (copol or a synthetic resin dissolved in an organic solvent such as acetone, chloroform or ether) and calcium hydroxide (calcium hydroxide and a solvent or hardener). Because cavity var-

nish contains many chemicals which may cause adverse reactions, it should be avoided. Calcium hydroxide is a more suitable pulp protector. Glass ionomer cements also make good cavity liners.

10) *Composite Filling Material*—As I discussed in the last chapter, composite filling materials are suitable for use as replacement materials in a good many circumstances. Their allergic potential should be evaluated.

## 3. ADDITIONAL FACTORS TO CONSIDER

1) *Testing of Dental Materials*—Testing of dental materials prior to their use is recommended by many clinical ecologists. If your physician believes that it is necessary to test the new materials, you should complete testing prior to beginning replacement procedures. It is important to note: if you don't have an adverse reaction to the tested dental materials, it is not a guarantee that you won't react to them in the future. If, however, you have followed the recommended treatment (diet, immunotherapy, etc.), you will have the best chance for improvement. I don't know of anyone who was "cured" by only replacing their amalgam fillings.

2) *Supplements*—Your physician should advise you as to which supplements to take. Most vitamin companies now list the ingredients, additives and the food source of their vitamins.

3) *Excretion of Mercury*—Once your amalgam fillings have been removed, some dentists and physicians suggest that you monitor the release of mercury from your cells and the excretion of this mercury from your body. This can be accomplished by 24-hour urine mercury levels. The most ideal circumstances allow your body to rid itself of mercury. If your body is not able to detoxify itself, the next step may be to supplement with specific nutrients, such as selenium, which have the ability to remove heavy metals. If supplementation proves not to be effective, drug therapy, such as penicillamine, may be indicated. Your physician should monitor your progress in this important area.

## LOOKING BACK

1. Allergy and EI patients must evaluate all dental chemicals and dental materials.
2. Allergy and EI patients should try to avoid as many dental chemicals as possible.

3. It is important to be medically stable prior to having your amalgam fillings replaced.
4. The use of a rubber dam and high-speed suction are necessary in removing amalgam fillings.
5. Gold is the superior filling material. Both the content of the gold product and the cements used to hold the filling in place should be evaluated before treatment begins.
6. You can have gold, composite and porcelain fillings in your mouth at the same time, but you should not have both gold and amalgam fillings in your mouth at the same time.
7. Some dental procedures which cause symptoms cannot be avoided, while others can.

## REFERENCES

1. Zamm, A.: *Mercury and Dentistry*, Kingston, New York, 1985.

# APPENDIX I

## QUICK-REFERENCE GLOSSARY

ACUTE—having a sudden onset, sharp rise, and short course.

AEROBIC—occurring only in the presence of oxygen.

ALLERGY—exaggerated or pathological reaction (as by sneezing, respiratory embarrassment, itching or skin rashes) to substances, situations, or physical states that are without comparable effect on the average individual.

ALLOY—a substance composed of two or more metals.

AMALGAM—an alloy of mercury with another metal that is solid or liquid at room temperature according to the proportion of mercury present.

AMALGAMATION—the process of combining mercury with a metal or an alloy to form a new alloy.

AMALGAMETER—the instrument used to measure the electric currents generated by amalgam fillings.

AMERICAN ACADEMY OF ENVIRONMENTAL MEDICINE—is a professional association consisting of physicians, dentists and other allied health professionals which has as its goal the identification and control of substances in a patient's environment that are causing his/her adverse reactions.

AMINO ACIDS—the chief components of protein which are synthesized by living cells or are obtained as essential components of the diet.

ANAEROBIC—occurring in the absence of oxygen.

ANEMIA—a condition in which the blood is deficient in red blood cells, in hemoglobin, or in total volume.

ANGINA—a disease marked by spasmodic attacks of severe pain in the chest usually caused by coronary disease.

ANTIBODIES—a specific protein produced by the body in response to an antigen.

ANTIGEN—a protein or carbohydrate substance (as a toxin or enzyme) that when introduced into the body stimulates the production of an antibody.

ASSIMILATION—the incorporation of digested materials from food, into the tissues of an organism.

ATAXIA—the inability to coordinate the muscles in the execution of voluntary movement.

ATELECTASIS—absence of gas (oxygen) from a part of the whole of the lungs, due to failure of expansion or resorption of gas.

AUTOIMMUNE DISEASE—a disease characterized by the condition in which one's own tissues are subject to deleterious effects of the immunological system.

B LYMPHOCYTE—a specialized white blood cell which produces antibodies

B-CELL—is a B lymphocyte.

BATTERY EFFECT—is the production of electric currents by metallic fillings due to the different electrical potentials of the various metals.

BINDING—the combining of two or more substances (as by chemical forces) to produce a new substance.

BIOCHEMICAL—characterized by, produced by, or involving chemical reactions in living organisms.

CANDIDA—an infection due to the fungus (Candida albicans) which is ordinarily a part of man's normal gastrointestinal flora, but which becomes pathogenic when there is a disturbance in the balance of that flora, e.g. from treatment with an antibiotic, or in debilitation of the host from other causes (cancer, diabetes).

CARBOHYDRATE—any of the various neutral compounds of carbon, hydrogen and oxygen (as sugars, starches and celluloses) most of which are formed by green plants and which constitute a major class of animal foods.

CELL—a minute structure, the living, active basis of all plant and animal organization.

CELL-MEDIATED IMMUNITY—immunity characterized by T-cells which have been sensitized to an antigen.

CHOREA—irregular, spasmodic, involuntary movements of the limbs or facial muscles.

CHRONIC—denoting a disease of slow progress and long duration.

COENZYME—a "helper" enzyme.

COENZYME A—A coenzyme that occurs in all living cells and is essential to the metabolism of carbohydrates, fats and some amino acids.

COLITIS—inflammation of the colon.

COLLAGEN DISEASE—is a term applied to diseases which involve the connective tissue system; examples are lupus erythematosus, scleroderma and rheumatoid arthritis.

COMPLEMENT—a protein complex found in blood serum. It aids in the destruction of foreign materials.

COMPOSITE—refers to a group of dental materials consisting of single organic chemicals (monomers) which join together to form large molecules (polymers) and fillers. These are a plastic-type filling material.

CONDENSATION—the process of packing a filling material, particularly amalgam, into a cavity, using such force and direction that excess mercury is expressed from the filling mass and no voids result.

CORROSION—the gradual deterioration of a substance by biochemical or chemical reaction.

CROWN—is a dental restoration (filling) which covers the entire tooth. This is usually made of gold, porcelain or a combination of gold and porcelain. Crowns are also referred to as "caps" or "jackets."

CYANOSIS—a dark bluish or purplish coloration of the skin and mucous membrane due to a deficiency of oxygen in the blood.

CYSTEINE—an amino acid found in most proteins.

CYTOTOXIC—a substance which is detrimental or destructive to cells.

DENTAL AMALGAM—a dental filling material consisting of mercury, silver, copper, tin and sometimes zinc.

DENTAL PULP—the soft tissue in the pulp cavity, consisting of connective tissue containing blood vessels, nerves and lymphatics.

DENTAL TUBULE—the channels containing nerves that are located in the dentin of the tooth.

DERMATITIS—inflammation of the skin.

DEVITALIZATION—the process by which the pulp is destroyed. This can occur by chemicals, infection or from the heat produced during a dental procedure.

DISULFIDE GROUP—(−SS) a group consisting of two sulfur atoms which are in combination with other atoms in a molecule.

DYCAL—a cavity lining material, consisting of calcium hydroxide, used for the protection of the pulp.

DYSFUNCTION—difficult to abnormal function.

EMPHYSEMA—a condition of the lung marked by expansion and frequently by impairment of heart action.

ENDODONTIC—a term referring to the biology and pathology of the dental pulp.

ENVIRONMENTAL ILLNESS—a disease characterized by acute adverse reactions to environmental substances.

ENZYME—a protein, secreted by cells, that acts as a catalyst to bring about chemical changes in other substances, itself remaining apparently unchanged by the process.

EPILEPSY—any of the various disorders marked by disturbed electrical rhythms of the central nervous system and typically manifested by convulsions usually with some alteration of consciousness.

ERYTHEMA—inflammatory redness of the skin.

ERYTHISM—a condition marked by exceptional prevalence of red pigmentation (as in skin or hair).

ESSENTIAL—necessary and indispensible; refers to those nutrients which are required for normal health and growth and cannot be manufactured by the body.

FAT—a greasy, soft-solid material, found in animal tissues and many plants.

FATTY ACID—is the individual component of fats, oils and waxes.

FOREIGN—a substance found in the living organism which is not a part of that organism.

GI TRACT—is the gastrointestional tract consisting of the stomach, intestines and colon.

GINGIVAL TISSUE—the soft tissue surrounding the tooth; sometimes referred to as the "gums."

GLUTATHIONE—a peptide (containing glutamic acid, cysteine, glycine) that occurs in plant and animal tissues and plays an important role in the activation of some enzymes.

GLYCOGEN—the principal carbohydrate reserve that is readily converted into glucose.

GRAM—a unit of weight equal to 1/1,000th kilogram.

HALF-TIME—the time for half of the substance to disappear.

H.E.A.L.—The Human Ecology Action League—a lay publication which has as its purpose, the collection and dissemination of information on environmental illness to persons suffering from that illness.

HEAVY METALS—any of a group of metals (mercury, lead and cadmium) with a high molecular weight and characterized by their ability to produce toxic reactions in living organisms.

HEMATOCRIT—the percentage of the volume of a blood sample occupied by cells.

HEMOGLOBIN—the red, respiratory protein of the red blood cells.

HISTAMINE—an organic compound, present in animal tissues, which plays a role in an allergic reaction. Histamine dilates blood vessels and increases cell permeability.

HORMONES—a product of living cells that circulates in body fluids and produces a specific effect on the activity of cells remote from its point of origin.

HUMORAL IMMUNITY—immunity associated with circulating antibodies.

HYPERGLYCEMIA—an abnormally high concentration of glucose in the circulating blood.

HYPOGLYCEMIA—an abnormally small concentration of glucose in the circulating blood.

HYPOPROTEINEMIA—abnormally small amounts of total protein in the circulating blood plasma.

IMMUNE COMPLEX—a combination of antigens and antibodies.

IMMUNOGLOBULIN—an immune protein made up of light and heavy chains of amino acids held together by disulfide bonds.

INFLAMMATION—a local response to cellular injury that is marked by redness, heat and pain.

INLAY—a pre-formed filling cemented into place which does not include the tips of the cusps of the tooth.

INORGANIC—an atom, molecule or compound not formed by a living organism.

INVERTASE—an enzyme capable of inverting the sugar, sucrose.

ION—an atom or group of atoms carrying a charge of electricity by virtue of having gained or lost one or more valence electrons.

LETHARGY—abnormal drowsiness.

LEUKOCYTE—white blood cell.

LICHEN PLANUS—eruption of flat-topped, shiny, papules on flexor surfaces.

LIGANDS—an organic molecule attached to a central metal ion by multiple coordination bonds.

LUPUS ERYTHEMATOSUS—one of the connective tissue diseases characterized by skin lesions.

LYMPH NODE—one of the rounded masses of lymphoid tissue surrounded by a capsule of connective tissue.

LYMPHOBLASTS—a young, immature cell which matures into a lymphocyte.

LYMPHOCYTE—a white blood cell formed throughout the body in lymph nodes, spleen, thymus, tonsils and sometimes in bone marrow.

LYMPHOKINES—soluble substances, released by sensitized lymphocytes on contact with specific antigen, which help effect cellular immunity by stimulating activity of monocytes and macrophages.

LYSIS—a process of disintegration of dissolution of cells, bacteria or antigens.

MACROPHAGES—a white blood cell which is responsible for presenting antigen to antibody-producing cells and aids in the destruction of foreign materials.

MEMBRANE PERMEABILITY—permitting the passage of substances through a membrane.

MERCURY—a heavy silver-white poisonous metallic element that is liquid at room temperatures.

METABOLISM—the sum of the chemical changes in living cells by which energy is provided for vital processes and activities and new material is assimilated to repair the waste.

MICROGRAM—(ug) one-millionth of a gram.

MILLIGRAM—(mg) one-thousandth of a gram.

MONOSACCHARIDES—a simple sugar which cannot be decomposed into simple sugars.

MULTIPLE SCLEROSIS—(MS) a diseased condition marked by patches of hardened tissue in the brain or spinal cord, causing some degree of paralysis, tremor, and disturbances of speech.

NAUSEA—a stomach distress with distaste for food and an urge to vomit.

NECROSIS—localized death of one or more cells, a portion of tissue or organ.

NEPHRITIS—inflammation of the kidneys.

NIOSH—National Institute of Occupational Safety and Health.

NON-ESSENTIAL—necessary and indispensible; refers to those nutrients which are required for normal health and growth and can be manufactured by the body.

NON-SELF—refers to compounds, cells, tissues or organs which are not a part of the living organism.

ONLAY—a filling which includes the tips of the cusps of the tooth.

ORGAN—any part of the body exercising a specific function, such as respiration, secretion or digestion.

ORGANIC—an atom, molecule or compound which is formed by a living organism.

OSHA—Occupational Safety and Health Administration.

PHAGOCYTOSIS—the process of ingestion and digestion by cells of solid substances, such as other cells, bacteria and foreign particles.

PLACENTA—the vascular organ of exchange between the fetus and the mother.

PNEUMOTHORAX—the presence of air or gas in the pleural cavity.

POISON—a substance which through its chemical action usually kills, injures or impairs an organism.

POLYNEUROPATHY—a disease process involving a number of peripheral nerves.

POLYPEPTIDE—a molecular chain of amino acids.

PROPHYLACTIC—tending to prevent disease.

PROSTHETIC DEVICE—a fabricated substitute for a diseased or missing part of the body, such as a limb, tooth, eye or heart valve.

PROSTODONTIST—a dentist who specializes in the replacement of missing or diseased teeth using gold fillings such as crowns, inlays or onlays.

PROTEIN—molecules consisting of long sequences of amino acids.

PROTEINURIA—the presence of urinary protein in concentrations greater than 0.3 g in a 24-hour urine collection.

PULP—the soft tissue in the pulp cavity, consisting of connective tissue containing blood vessels, nerves and lymphatics.

QUADRANT—a quarter of a circle. The teeth are envisioned to be in a circle with the chewing surface on the horizontal plane and the left and right sides divided in half by the vertical plane.

REMISSION—abatement or lessening in severity of the symptoms of the disease.

RESPIRATION—the exchange of oxygen and carbon dioxide that occurs within an individual cell, tissue, organ and organism.

RESTORATIONS—any substance such as gold, amalgam, composite, etc. used for restoring the portion missing from a tooth as a result of drilling out decay in the tooth.

RUBBER DAM—a thin square piece (4.5 inches) of rubber used to isolate the tooth from the mouth.

SCLERODERMA—a disease of the skin characterized by thickening and hardening of the subcutaneous tissues.

SELF—a compound, cell, tissue or organ which is a part of the organism.

SINUSITIS—inflammation of the lining membrane of the sinus.

SODIUM ASCORBATE—same action and uses of ascorbic acid; it is preferred for intramuscular administration.

SPLEEN—a highly vascular ductless organ near the stomach concerned with final destruction of blood cells, storage of blood and production of lymphocytes.

STOMATITIS—inflammation of the mucous membrane of the mouth.

SULFHYDRYL GROUP—(−SH) a group consisting of a hydrogen and a sulfur atom which are in combination with other atoms in a molecule.

T LYMPHOCYTE—a white cell which is responsible for the regulation of antibody formation by other white blood cells.

T-CELLS—T lymphocytes.

TACHYCARDIA—rapid heart beating.

TACHYPNEA—rapid breathing.

THYMUS GLAND—glandular structure that is necessary in early life for the normal development of immunologic function.

TISSUE—a collection of similar cells.

TLV—Threshold Limit Value.

TOXIN—a noxious or poisonous substance.

TREMOR—an involuntary trembling movement.


UNIVERSAL REACTOR—is a patient who reacts adversely to many substances in their environment not known to cause reactions in other individuals.

UREASE—an enzyme that promotes the hydrolysis of urea.

URINALYSIS—is the analysis of the urine.


WHITE BLOOD CELL—a blood cell which is responsible for defense.


Compiled from *Webster's New World Dictionary*, G. and C. Merriam Co. and *Stedman's Medical Dictionary*, Williams and Wilkins.

# APPENDIX TWO

## GOVERNMENT SAFETY STANDARDS
### By Terri Skladany Fasciana, M.S., J.D.

A common question raised by anyone who is exposed to toxins or chemicals is "how much will it hurt me?" To answer that question, you should know what degree of exposure is considered safe and how that safe level is determined. The purpose of this appendix is to inform you about the relevant government safety standards established for use in the workplace. The discussion focuses on the standard established for mercury by the Occupational Safety and Health Administration (OSHA). This appendix also raises concerns about blind reliance on standards and how confident we can be that strict adherence to them will protect our good health.

## 1. CONGRESS ESTABLISHES OSHA AND NIOSH

In 1970 Congress passed the Occupational Safety and Health Act which created both OSHA (Occupational Safety and Health Administration) and NIOSH (National Institute for Occupational Safety and Health).[1] This Act (statute) set specific goals and explicitly delegated authority to each agency. The power delegated to OSHA and NIOSH reflects the goals and purposes assigned to each. This discussion concentrates on the agency's task of evaluating safe standards for chemical and toxic exposure in the workplace.

### A. OSHA

OSHA was created within the Labor Department and was given the authority to set and enforce federal health and safety standards in order to protect approximately fifty-five million industrial, farm and commercial workers. The agency is authorized to inspect the workplace, to require employers to keep account of worker injury and illness, and to conduct research. OSHA is also empowered to issue standards for acceptable exposure limits to toxic chemicals and hazardous substances. Within one month after its inception, OSHA adopted 4,400 standards from existing federal regulations, industry codes and the National Standards Institute.[2] The TLV for mercury was one of these adopted standards. OSHA adopted the TLV for mercury as a consensus standard. This consensus standard was taken from the levels of mercury accepted as safe by the American Conference for government and Industrial Hygienists and the American National Standard Institute. The present OSHA standard for mercury is 50 ug/m$^3$. The measurement is the maximum exposure to mercury vapor that is not harmful over a series of five daily exposure periods of eight hours each during a one-week interval.

### B. NIOSH

On the other hand, NIOSH was created under the Department of Health, Education and Welfare to conduct job safety research. Its purpose is to investigate toxic chemicals, hazardous wastes, etc. and to recommend the levels of exposure which it believes are acceptable. Its goal is to protect the health and the welfare of workers. You should be aware that NIOSH has no authority to set acceptable levels of chemicals in the workplace—its role is merely advisory. NIOSH has recommended an acceptable TLV for mercury as 20 ug/m$^3$, which is less than half of the level of mercury exposure that is presently acceptable according to OSHA standards.

## 2. THE DECISION ABOUT STANDARDS

### A. Setting Agency Rules

In cases where an agency does not adopt a consensus standard, it may be important for you to have an awareness of the usual procedures that an agency must follow when it adopts rules or standards to better understand the proper role of a standard in protecting the public safety. The procedures are initially set by Congress in the statute which creates the agency. In this "organic statute," Congress sets the policies which it wants the agency to follow, and it calls for either formal rule making or informal rule making. Once the organic statute "triggers" either formal or informal rule making, then the agency must follow the steps established in the Administrative Procedure Act.

Formal rule making requires a full adjudicative hearing before the rule goes into effect.[3] What this means is that the agency's rule must be based solely on the information in the record which was compiled at the hearing. This data would include scientific evidence and the testimony of expert witnesses. In formal rule making, the agency acts like a court—it is an adversary proceeding with witnesses, cross examination, etc. Once the hearing is completed, the agency then issues a written opinion that makes findings and conclusions based only on the information presented at the hearing.

However, this type of formal rule making is rarely required by

Congress. Usually, Congress calls for only informal rule making.[4] Informal rule making is also known as "notice and comment" because of the relaxed procedures that the agency follows in formulating the rule. Informal rule making involves six steps:

1. *Notice of the Proposed Rule in the Federal Register*—The chairman of the agency places a notice in the Federal Register. This notice sets out the proposed rule, tells the public what is involved and invites written comment. The agency must give the public a reasonable time to submit its comments, usually 30 days.

2. *Written Comment*—Once written comments are received the agency will consider any relevant material which is submitted. However, the agency is not bound to use any of the written material received when it makes its final decision.

3. *Agency Consideration*—In informal rule making, the agency is not restricted in considering only the information in the written comment. It may take into account any information which it feels is applicable. The agency is acting like a legislature—it receives and acts on the viewpoints and data without a trial type of procedure. The agency decision is only based on the information which it sees fit to include in the record. Therefore, interested parties usually do not have a significant chance to participate in the decision.

4. *Final Rule*—The final agency rule is then placed in the Federal Register. This notice will include the statement of the rule, its basis and purpose.

5. *Effective Date*—Once the final rule is published, at least thirty days must pass before the rule goes into effect. This second notice serves two purposes: it gives the public notice as to what the rule requires and it announces the possible sanctions if the rule is not followed.

6. *Judicial Review*—Once the rule goes into effect, the courts must wait for an individual who is harmed by the rule to challenge it. Once a person who is harmed makes that challenge the court can hear the case based on what factors the injured party disputes.

### B. Challenging an Agency Rule

As you have seen, OSHA is not bound by the research of its own scientists or by standards recommended by NIOSH. However, if the substance of the standard or regulation adopted by OSHA is challenged in court, OSHA must show that the standard is supported by "substantial evidence."[5] The "substantial evidence" test means that the agency must demonstrate two things: that its decision has support through evidence it has compiled in the record and that there is a reasonable basis for the agency decision. If these two criteria are met, the agency standard will be upheld by the court.[6] In most instances, it is unlikely that the court will overturn the agency decision because the standard established by the agency is not supported by substantial evidence. The reasoning behind this policy is that since Congress created the agency as an expert in the area delegated to it, the court will defer to the agency expertise on all questions of fact. Therefore, most agency standards will be upheld.

### C. Understanding the Agency's Role

To put the agency's job of setting a standard for mercury exposure and other chemical exposures into perspective, I will briefly describe the purpose of the agency and the issues that one should evaluate when applying the "acceptable" standards for toxic chemicals and hazardous substances.

OSHA's major function is to set and enforce safety and health standards to protect workers in industry, agriculture and construction. Section 6 (b)(5) of the Occupational Safety and Health Act states that:

> The Secretary, in promulgating standards dealing with toxic materials or harmful physical agents under this subsection, shall set the standards which most adequately assure, to the extent feasible, on the basis of the best available evidence, that no employee will suffer material impairment of health or functional capacity even if such employee has regular exposure to the hazard dealt with by such standard for the period of his working life.[7]

As you can see, the statute focuses the agency on setting a standard which will protect employees from "material impairment" of health or functional capacity. This standard is a far cry from requiring a healthy work place or setting standards which promote good health.

Charles Schultz, a former Chairman of the President's Council of Economic Advisors, in an address at the Brookings Institution noted that:

The Federal Government has recently entered in a big way the field of regulating health and safety in the work place throughout the country. The complexities of controlling industrial accidents, and over the longer run the even greater problem of identifying and dealing with the industrial health problems in a chemically inventive society, are as great as those of energy and the environment.[8]

As you can see, OSHA's job is both substantial and complex when you consider just how "chemically inventive" industry and farming have become within the past ten years. In addition to the complexity of OSHA's job, there are additional factors which you should consider when you appraise the proper weight that should be given to the OSHA standard for mercury.

1. Scientific knowledge is limited—Since ethical principles prohibit testing toxic chemicals on humans, our knowledge of what mercury levels are "safe" must be interpreted from animal studies. Since animals are smaller and have a shorter life span than human beings, the animal data may not accurately indicate what effect long-term exposure to a substance such as mercury could have on a human being. Furthermore, animal experiment give us only objective, measurable data. Since the animal cannot report its symptoms to the researcher, our findings will be focused on only the effects of the toxin which can be documented through testing. The scientific conclusions do not address the subtle yet debilitating effects that toxins have on mood, energy, psychological outlook and general wellbeing.

2. Individuality—Animal studies indicating "acceptable" levels of exposure do not allow for individual human differences. The TLV for mercury does not and cannot evaluate the role that genetic factors, exposure to other harmful or toxic substances and lifestyle may play in determining what level of mercury is safe for you as an individual.

In conclusion, the OSHA standard for mercury is only a general guideline which was adopted in 1970 to prevent "material impairment of health" caused by exposure to harmful or toxic substances in the work place. This standard does not evaluate individual differences, genetic makeup, lifestyle or exposure to other chemicals and toxins. Therefore levels of exposure below the OSHA TLV are false guarantees that your exposure to mercury is acceptable because there can be no standard that is safe for everyone.

## REFERENCES

1. Occupational Safety and Health Act, 29 U.S.C. § 651 (1970).
2. Congressional Quarterly, Inc., *Regulation Process and Politics* (1982).
3. Administrative Procedure Act, 5 U.S.C. § 556, 557 (1966).
4. Administrative Procedure Act, 5 U.S.C. § 553 (1966).
5. Administrative Procedure Act, 5 U.S.C. § 706 (1966)
6. *National Labor Relations Board v. Hearst Publications, Inc.*, 322 U.S. 111, 88 L.Ed. 1170 (1944).
7. Occupational Safety and Health Act, 29 U.S.C. § 655(b) (5) (1970).
8. Gellhorn, W., Byse, C. and Strauss, P. L.: *Administrative Law* 2-5 (1979).

# APPENDIX THREE

## SURVEY LETTERS

# 1. SURVEY OF THE CLINICAL ECOLOGISTS

The following letter was sent to clinical ecologists believed to treat a sizable number of chemically sensitive patients in order to provide input from their experiences with amalgam replacement in patients having chemical sensitivities or acute allergies.

---

Guy S. Fasciana, D.M.D.
106 Naussau Drive
Springfield, Mass. 01129

January 9, 1985

Dear Doctor:

I write a column in *The Human Ecologist* entitled "The Ecological Dentist" which addresses the relationship between dental materials and environmental illness.

After writing a fairly comprehensive analysis of dental materials, I received quite a few letters asking me to dedicate a column to mercury and its relationship to environmental illness. I have contacted both the American Dental Association and the proponents of the "mercury replacement" school and am in need of some unbiased clinical data or experiences. I would like this article to be as objective and as helpful as possible, therefore I am soliciting your help. Many patients and Clinical Ecologists may be relying on the information and conclusion that I make on this subject. Both positive and negative feedback would be appreciated.

I would appreciate information on the following:
1. Have you had patients diagnosed as having EI?
2. If comprehensive treatment was accomplished, was one of the recommended procedures the replacement of silver amalgam fillings?
3. If filling replacment was recommended:
   a. Did replacement take place?
   b. Was the replacement successful?
   c. Relative to #2 above, when did replacement occur? (e.g., was it the first treatment tried, the last or in between?)

 d. What were the fillings replaced with?
 e. Is the patient having any difficulty with the new fillings?
 4. In your clinical experience, what roles do mercury and silver amalgam fillings play in EI?

I would very much appreciate your response in this matter.

Sincerely,
Guy S. Fasciana, D.M.D.

---

## 2. PRELIMINARY PATIENT SURVEY:

The following questions appeared as part of a survey published in *The Human Ecologist* (#27, Fall 1984).

1. Sex, age.
2. Are you sensitive to any of the following: chemicals, foods, molds, seasonals, dust, mites, Candida?
3. Have you ever been diagnosed as having hypoglycemia?
4. Do you have amalgam fillings? Gold fillings? Gum disease?
5. Do you have unusual tastes in your mouth?
6. Describe reactions to dental treatment.
7. Have you ever been advised to replace your amalgam fillings? If so, did you? Was the replacement successful? What materials were used to replace the amalgam fillings?

---

**3. PATIENT FOLLOW-UP LETTER**—to patients who indicated that they had had their amalgam fillings replaced:

---

Guy S. Fasciana, D.M.D.
106 Nassau Drive
Springfield, Mass. 01129

Dear Patient:

Thank you for filling out the dental survey which appeared in *The Human Ecologist*. I am still researching the mercury controversy and anticipate a report shortly. Below are some additional questions for those patients who have had their silver amalgam fillings replaced. Since I want the report to be as objective and complete as possible, I am asking for your input once again. If you have any friends who have had their amalgams replaced, I would appreciate hearing from them also. I am looking for both positive and negative results.

Thank you very much for your interest and cooperation.

Sincerely,
Guy S. Fasciana, D.M.D.

1. General health prior to treatment.
2. Signs and symptoms attributed to dental mercury.
3. Significant factors in history leading to diagnosis.
4. Objective tests performed which led to diagnosis.
5. If Patch test: brand, agent used, method.
6. If amalgameter: brand, use.
7. If hair analysis, blood or urine: lab test, results.
8. Vitamins, detox agents and digestive enzymes used: brand, dose
9. Was the replacement restorative material tested?
10. Time schedule from diagnosis to completion of treatment.
11. Ill effects (if any) during removal and thereafter.
12. Ill effects (if any) with new restorations.
13. What was the replacement restorative material?
14. What signs and symptoms were eliminated?
15. Physician's and dentist's name and address.
16. Could you make a chronological (month and year) list of the following: amalgam fillings, antibiotics, steroids, diagnosis of EI, avoidance of chemicals etc., allergy shots, diet changes, vitamin use, metabolic support, candida shots, nystatin, and filling replacements.

| Date | Event | Symptoms | Improvements |
|------|-------|----------|--------------|
|      |       |          |              |

## 4. SURVEY OF DENTISTS:

The following letter was sent to those dentists involved in the replacement of amalgams (names provided in clinical ecologists' survey).

Guy S. Fasciana, D.M.D.
106 Naussau Dr.
Springfield, Mass. 01129

March 22, 1985

Dear Doctor:

I am writing an article about the health implications of dental mercury. I would appreciate it if you could spend a few minutes to answer the enclosed questions. Your feedback is important to me.

Sincerely,
Guy S. Fasciana, D.M.D.

1. General health of patients prior to treatment.
2. Signs and symptoms present attributed to dental mercury.
3. Significant factors in the dental or medical history leading to diagnosis.
4. Objective tests performed which led to diagnosis.
5. If Patch test: brand, agent used, vehicle, protocol.
6. If amalgameter: brand, use.
7. If hair analysis, blood or urine: lab test, results.
8. Vitamins: brand, protocol.
9. Was the replacement restorative material tested?
10. Time schedule: general time frame from diagnosis to completion of treatment.
11. Ill effects (if any) during removal and thereafter.
12. Ill effects (if any) with new restorations.
13. What was the replacment restorative material?
14. What signs and symptoms were eliminated?
15. Approximate number of patients completed, percent success, reasons for failure.
16. Are you concerned about your own exposure to mercury?
17. Do you take any precautions to protect yourself from exposure?

## DENTAL MATERIALS

# 1. BACKGROUND

For many patients, the choice of dental materials used to replace their amalgam fillings is extremely important to whether they will be successful in achieving optimal health. The greater the patient's illness, the more important is this selection. For example, a selection which produces allergic reactions may reduce the benefits of replacing amalgam fillings.

As you have seen, there are numerous dental products each of which contains a variety of substances. Amalgam fillings contain several metals, dentures contain several chemicals and pigments and so on. Within a family of dental products (e.g., composites), there are many similar substances. In that same family, products from various manufacturers also contain distinct substances. For example, two composite filling materials may differ only in the "fillers" that they contain. If the filler of one manufacturer's composite contains something that you are allergic to or something that could cause a toxic reaction, that material will have to be avoided. For example, Trans-Lit (Merz + Co.) composite contains fillers made from oyster shells and contains 0.02 percent mercury-amidochloride.

An intelligent approach to dental materials is to eliminate those materials with which you know you have a problem. Next, evaluate the remaining materials for potential problems by examining the ingredients and then, if necessary, to test the material for sensitivity reactions. Your physician will help you with this step. It is very important to note that filling materials do vary from time to time because a manufacturer may not be committed to using each specific ingredient. They may substitute ingredients according to availability of those ingredients. This occurs to a greater extent in generic dental materials.

Another shortcoming in evaluating a dental material is that dental manufacturers may not disclose all ingredients of their products to the general public because of market competition and trademark and patent considerations. In this case the manufacturer may have informed the Food and Drug Administration and/or the ADA of the contents of the individual dental materials; while some of the specific ingredients and percentages of those listed ingredients are privileged information. In the final analysis, if you are a highly allergic individual, you may need to test each dental material that you are going to use prior to beginning treatment.

This section discusses some of the more popular dental materials used in the replacement of amalgam fillings and lists those ingredients and percentages that I have been able to obtain from the literature produced by the manufacturer and/or direct correspondence with the manufacturers. Some manufacturers are more cooperative in disclosing the contents of their products. This list is not meant to be all inclusive; there are other dental materials which you may want to consider and there are new materials introduced to the dental market fairly frequently.

## 2. INTRODUCTION TO DENTAL MATERIALS

Gold alloys contain several of the following metals: gold, platinum, palladium, copper, silver, zinc, tin, iridium and indium. The gold alloy list contains the popular gold alloys which contain a high nobel metal content (gold, platinum and palladium). Please note that palladium has produced some adverse reactions in patients, copper is an immunosuppressant and there may be other trace metals not disclosed by the manufacturer.

Porcelain products, and a relatively new material, "cast glass," are used for full crowns (caps) in the front and back teeth. Manufacturers report that porcelain is "inert"; that is, no substances are given off by the material.

Composite filling materials contain many different chemicals, fillers and pigments. The composite filling materials recommended by dental manufacturers for use in the posterior (back) teeth are listed along with their ingredients.

There are two types of temporary cements: eugenol and eugenol-free. Since many allergy patients have reactions to eugenol (oil of cloves), the eugenol-free material may be indicated. Nogenol (Coe Company) is such a temporary cement whose main ingredients are zinc undecylenate, peanut oil and peppermint oil.

Permanent cements include zinc phosphate, zinc silicophosphate, EBA zinc polyacrylate and glass ionomer. These cements may contain the ingredients listed but, may have additional ingredients as well.

Pulp protection is accomplished by calcium hydroxide bases which generally contain calcium tungstate, tribasic calcium phosphate and zinc oxide in glycol salicylate. The catalyst is calcium hydroxide, zinc oxide and zinc stearate in ethylene toluene sulfonamide. There may be other ingredients as well. Glass ionomer cements may also be used.

**GOLD ALLOYS**

| Brand | Company | Gold Type | Gold | Platinum | Composition (%) Palladium | Silver | Copper | Zinc |
|---|---|---|---|---|---|---|---|---|
| Modulay | Jelenko | II | 77 | — | 1 | 14 | — | — |
| Jel-2 | Jelenko | II | 71 | — | 2.5 | 17 | — | — |
| Firmilay | Jelenko | III | 74.5 | — | 3.5 | 11 | — | — |
| Jelenko-7 | Jelenko | IV | 69 | 3 | 3.5 | 12.5 | — | — |
| Jelenko-0 | Jelenko | IV | 87.5 | 4.5 | 6 | 1 | — | — |
| ORO A-1 | Ney | II | 78 | — | 2 | 12 | 7 | 1 |
| ORO B02 | NEY | III | 74 | — | 4 | 11.5 | 9.5 | 1 |
| ORO G-3 | Ney | IV | 69 | 3 | 4 | 12 | 11 | 2 |
| ORO 5 | Ney | IV | 63 | — | 5 | 19 | 12 | — |
| Bio-C | APM Stern | III | 80 | 18.85 | — | — | — | — |
| Bio-H | APM Stern | IV | 70 | 5 | — | 8 | <15 | — |
| Harmony Medium | Williams | II | 77 | — | 1 | 13 | 8.5 | — |
| Hard | | III | 74 | — | 4 | 12 | 9 | — |

# PORCELAIN

| Brand | Manufacturer | Contents |
|---|---|---|
| Cerestore | J&J | Unavailable |
| Ceramco | J&J | Unavailable |

## COMPOSITE FILLING MATERIALS

| | |
|---|---|
| COMPOSITE: | P30* |
| MANUFACTURER: | 3M |
| MONOMER: | BIS-GMA |
| | (2,2-bis[4(2-hydroxy-3 methacryloyloxy-propyloxy)-phenyl]propane) |
| FILLER: | Barium glass; zinc glass |
| DILUENT: | TEGDMA (triethyleneglycol dimethacrylate) |
| INHIBITOR: | Phenolic compounds |
| PIGMENTS: | Iron oxide; titanium dioxide |
| | *P30 also contains aluminum |

| | |
|---|---|
| COMPOSITE: | FulFil |
| MANUFACTURER: | L.D. Caulk |
| MONOMER: | BIS-GMA |
| FILLER: | Barium glass (76%); aluminum silicate (2%) |
| DILUENT: | Methyl methacrylate |
| INHIBITOR: | Alpha diketone |
| PIGMENTS: | Iron oxide; titanium oxide and channel black |

| COMPOSITE: | Sinterfil |
|---|---|
| MANUFACTURER: | Teledyne-Getz |
| MONOMER: | BIS-GMA; Urethane dimethacrylate |
| FILLER: | Colloidal silica; barium glass |
| DILUENT: | TEGDMA |
| INHIBITOR: | BHT (butylated hydroxytoluene) |
| PIGMENTS: | Titanium dioxide; chromium dioxide |

| COMPOSITE: | Occlusin |
|---|---|
| MANUFACTURER: | Coe |
| MONOMER: | Urethane dimethacrylate |
| FILLER: | Barium glass |
| DILUENT: | Urethane dimethacrylate |
| INHIBITOR: | Hydroquinine |
| PIGMENTS: | None |

| COMPOSITE: | SR-Isosit-N |
|---|---|
| MANUFACTURER: | Ivoclar |
| MONOMER: | Urethane dimethacrylate |
| FILLER: | Aerofil (silicon dioxide) |
| DILUENT: | None |
| INHIBITOR: | None |
| PIGMENTS: | Unavailable |

# PERMANENT CEMENTS

## 1. ZINC PHOSPHATE CEMENTS

*Contents:*

Zinc oxide
Magnesium oxide
Silicon dioxide
Bismuth trioxide
Ortho phosphoric acid

*Pigments:*

Copper oxide
Manganese dioxide
Platinum black
Powdered charcoal
Bismuth oxide
Titanium compounds
Alumunum

*Brands:*

Fleck's Cement (Mizzy)
Zinc Cement (S.S. White)
Ames C&B (Teledyne-Getz)

## 2. ZINC SILICOPHOSPHATE CEMENTS

*Contents:*

Contains ingredients
of zinc phosphate
cements with the addition
of silicate powders.

*Brands:*

Fluorothin (S.S. White)
Lucent (L.D. Caulk)
Dorcate (L.D. Caulk)

## 3. ZINC POLYACRYLATE (ZINC POLYCARBOXYLATE) CEMENTS

*Contents:*

Polyacrylic acid
Sodium hydroxide
Itaconic acid
Tartaric acid
Zinc oxide
Magnesium oxide
Alumina

*Brands:*

PCA (S.S. White)
Duralon (Espe)
Ames Polycarboxylate (Teledyne-Getz)

## 4. GLASS IONOMER CEMENTS

*Contents:*

Polyacrylic acid
Itaconic acid
Calcium fluoroaluminosilicate glass
Tartaric acid

*Brands:*

Ketac-Cem (Espe)

G.C. lining cements (G.C. International

## SUGGESTED READINGS

"Clinical Products in Dentistry," *JADA*, 109:821–864, November 1984.

Cousins, N.: *Anatomy of an Illness*, Bantam Books, New York, 1979.

Crook, W.: *The Yeast Connection*, Professional Books, Jackson, Tennessee, 1983.

Dickey, L.: *Clinical Ecology*, Charles Thomas, Springfield, Ill., 1976.

Eggleston, D.: "Effect of Dental Amalgam and Nickel Alloys on T-lymphocytes: Preliminary report," *J Pros Dent*, 51(5):617–623, May 1984.

Fasciana, G.: *Dental Materials: An Outline for the Allergic and Chemically Sensitive Patient*, Fasciana, G., 106 Naussau Drive, Springfield, Massachusetts, 1983.
Fasciana, T.: "Spring Cleaning: You Don't Have to Pollute to Clean!" *Vegetarian Times*, May 1982, 41.

Hunter, B.: *Consumer Beware*, Simon and Schuster, New York, 1971.

Kroker, G., Marshall, R. and Randolph, T.: "Acrylic Denture Intolerance in Multiple Food and Chemical Sensitivity," *Clinical Ecology*, 1(1):48–52, Spring 1982.

Levin, A. and Dadd, D.: *A Consumer Guide for the Chemically Sensitive*, Levin, A., San Francisco, 1982.

O'Brien, W. and Ryge, G.: *An Outline of Dental Materials*, W.B. Saunders, Philadelphia, 1978.

Nazzaro, A. and Lombard, D.: *The PMS Solution*, Winston Press, Minneapolis, 1985.

Philpott, W. and Kalita, D.: *Brain Allergies: The Psychonutrient Connection*, Keats Press, New Canaan, Connecticut, 1980.

Randolph, T. and Moss, R.: *An Alternative Approach to Allergies*, Lippincott and Crowell, New York, 1979.

Saifer, P. and Zellerbach, M.: *Detox*, Houghton Mifflin, Los Angeles, 1984.

Simonton, O., Matthews-Simonton, S. and Creighton, J.: *Getting Well Again*, Bantam Books, New York, 1978.

Störtebecker, P., M.D., Ph.D.: *Mercury Poisoning from Dental Amalgam— A Hazard to the Human Brain*, Störtebecker Foundation, Åkerbyuägen 282, S-183 35 Täby/Stockholm, Sweden, 1986.

Trakhtenberg, I.: *Chronic Effects of Mercury on Organisms*, (Translation by Fogarty International Center for Advanced Study in the Health Sciences), U.S. Dept of HEW Public Service, National Institute of Health, D HEW Pub (NIH), 1974.

Truss, C.: *The Missing Diagnosis*, Truss, C., Birmingham, Ala., 1983.

Zamm, A. and Gannon, R.: *Why Your House May Endanger Your Health*, Simon and Schuster, New York, 1980.

Zamm, A.: *Mercury and Dentistry*, Kingston, New York, 1985.

## ABOUT THE AUTHOR . . .

Guy S. Fasciana received his Doctor of Dental Medicine Degree from the University of Pittsburgh in 1971. He practiced general dentistry in Wyoming, Pennsylvania for eight years when he learned that he was allergic to dental chemicals and dental materials. Since that time, he has researched what makes people ill (toxins, allergens, etc.) in dentistry and in the general environment.

Dr. Fasciana writes a column called "The EI Dentist" for *The Human Ecologist*, the environmental health magazine of the Human Ecology Action League (H.E.A.L.).

The professional organizations to which Dr. Fasciana is affiliated include the American Dental Association, the Pennsylvania Dental Society, and the American Academy of Environmental Medicine.

## OTHER PUBLICATIONS BY THE AUTHOR:

*Dental Materials: An Outline for the Allergic and Chemically Sensitive Patient*, Springfield, Massachusetts, 1985.

"Dental Materials—Part III," *The Human Ecologist*, 27:11-13, 1984.

"Dental Materials—Part II," *The Human Ecologist*, 26:11-12, 1984.

"Dental Materials—Part I," *The Human Ecologist*, 25:9-11, 1984.

"Choosing a Dentist," *The Human Ecologist*, 23:17-18, 1984.

"Food Allergy Provokes Myofacial Pain Dysfunction Symptoms," *Clinical Ecology*, vol. II, No. 1, pp. 21-26, (1983).

"Does Your Life-Style Prevent Disease or Prevent Health?," Wyoming, Pa., 1979.

"Have It My Way—A Successful Approach to Oral Health," Wyoming, Pa., 1975.

"A Successful Method for Optimum Oral Health," Wyoming, Pa., 1973.